Fungal Infection

Edited by Érico Silva de Loreto
and Juliana Simoni Moraes Tondolo

Published in London, United Kingdom

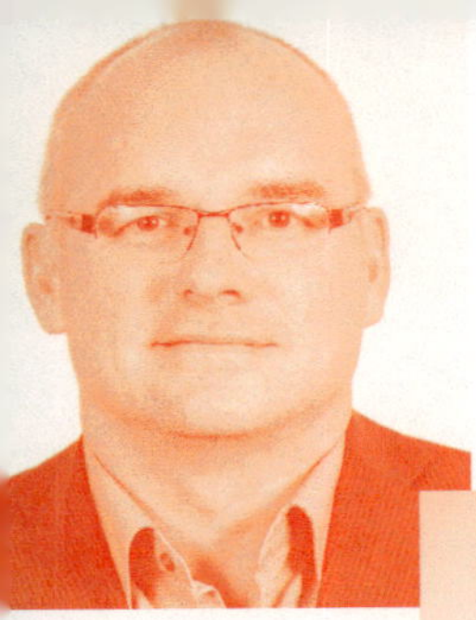
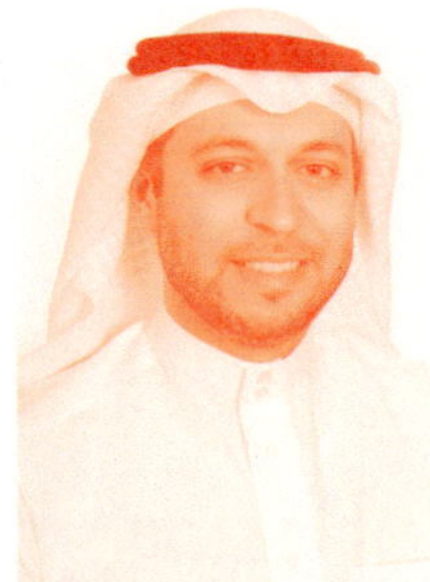
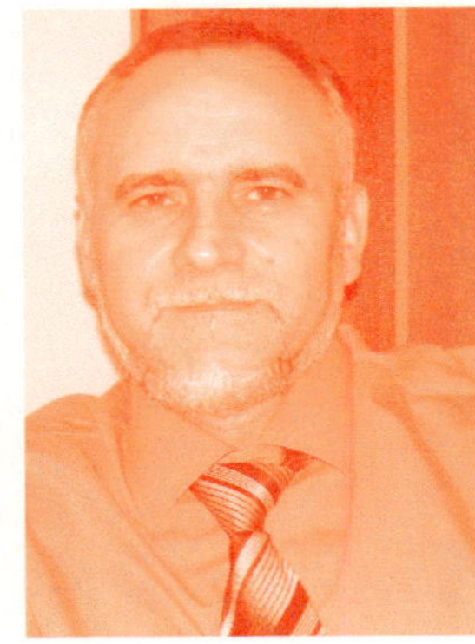
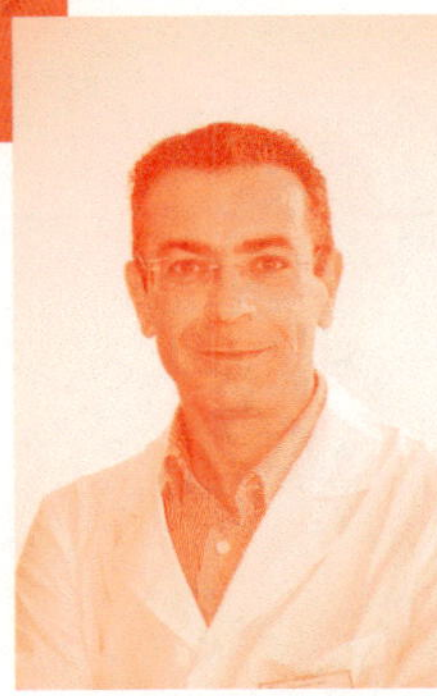
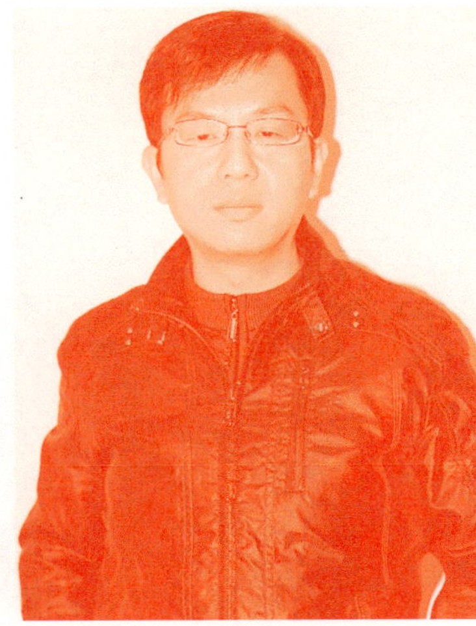
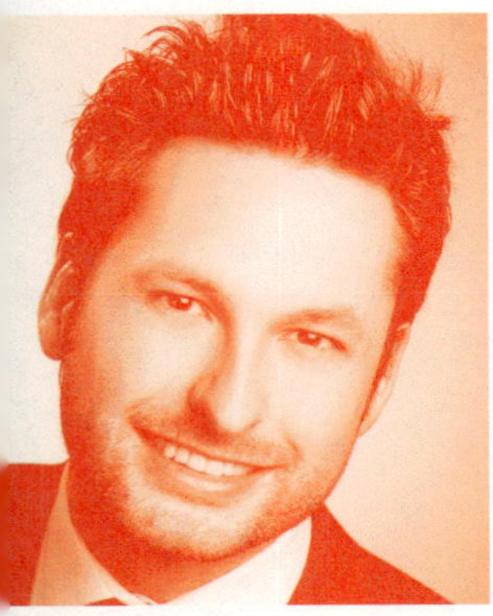
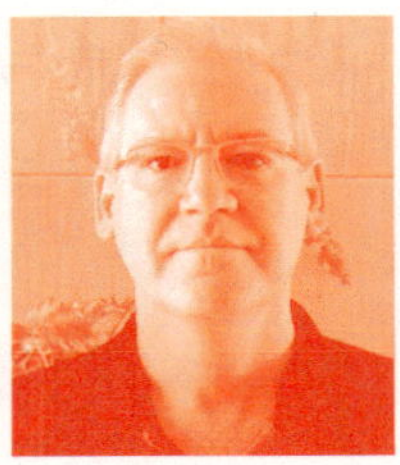

IntechOpen

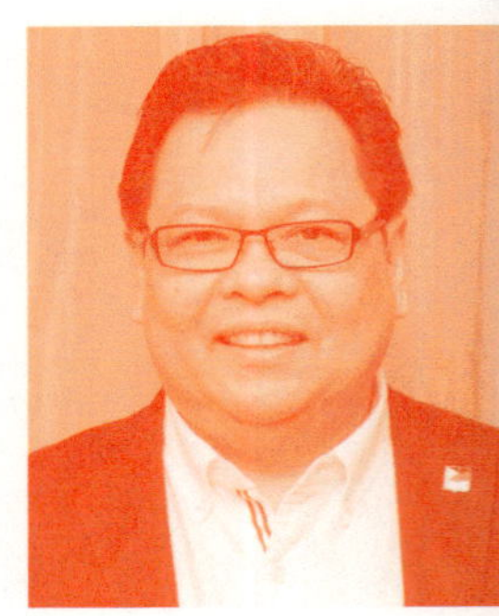
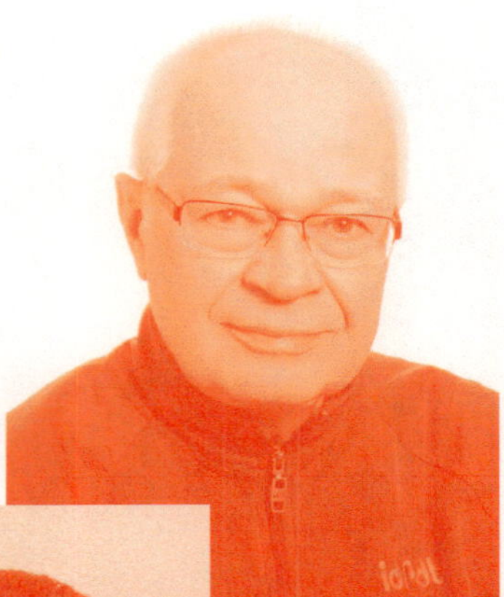
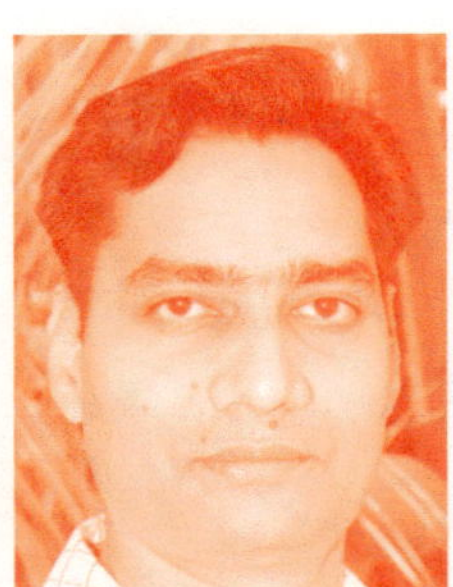
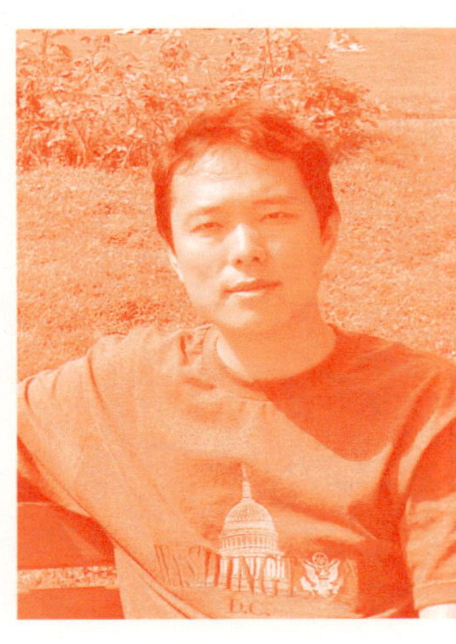
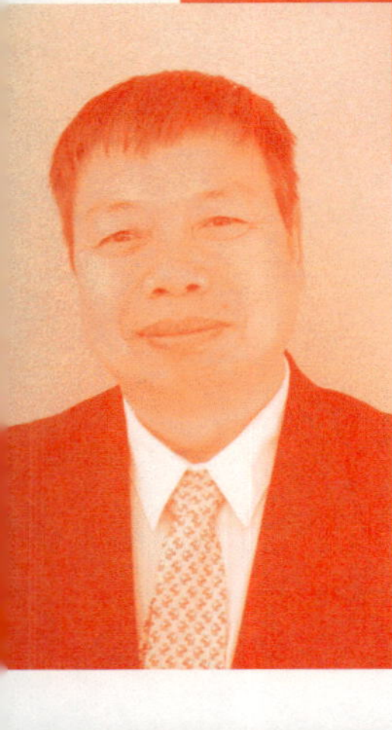
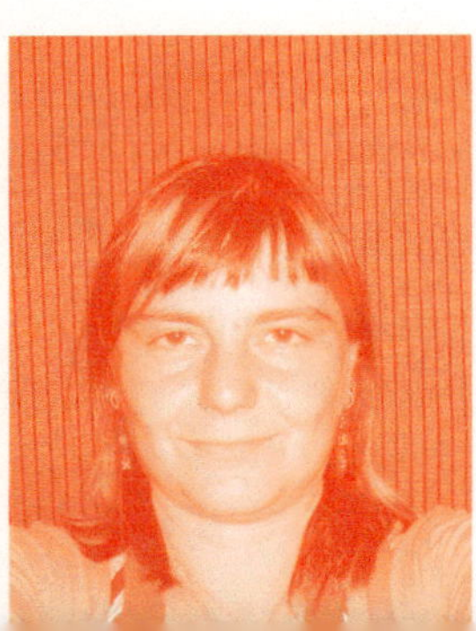

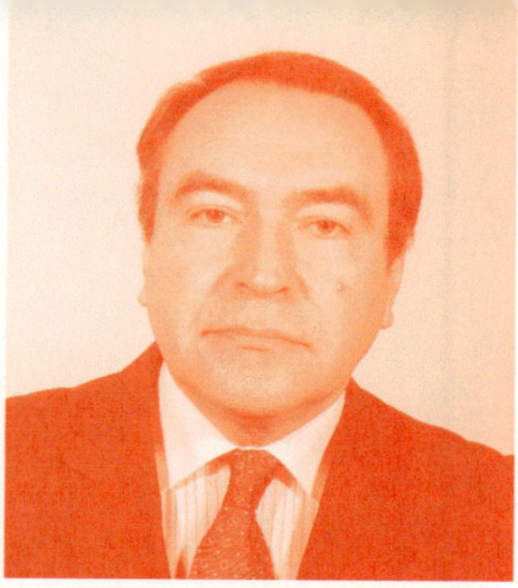
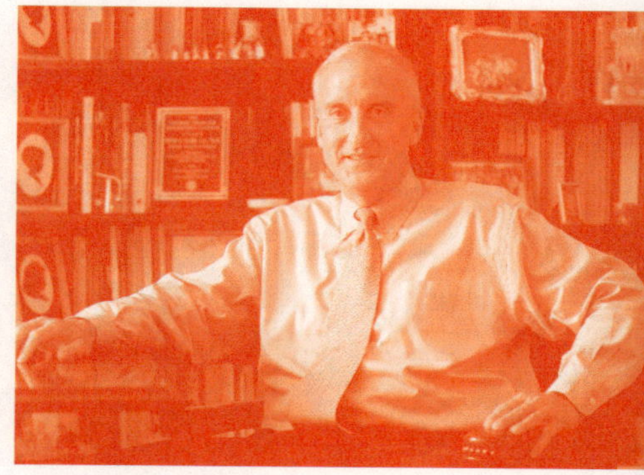
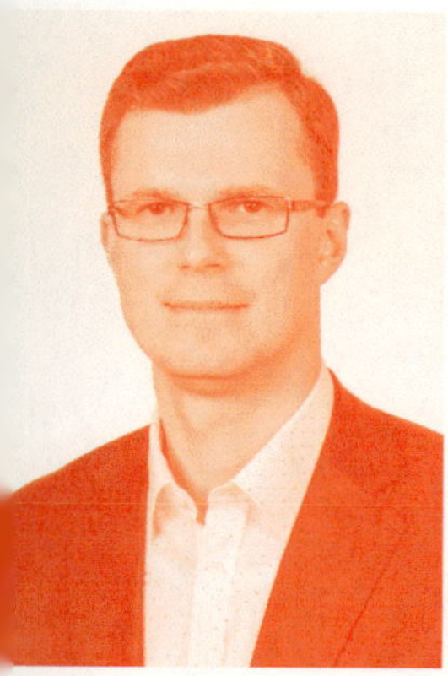
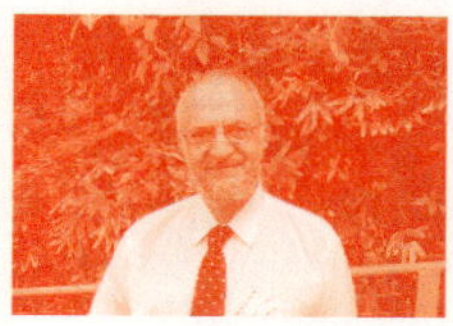
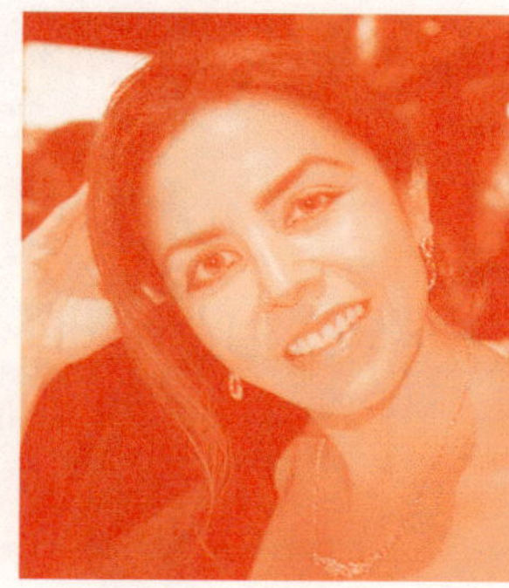

Supporting open minds since 2005

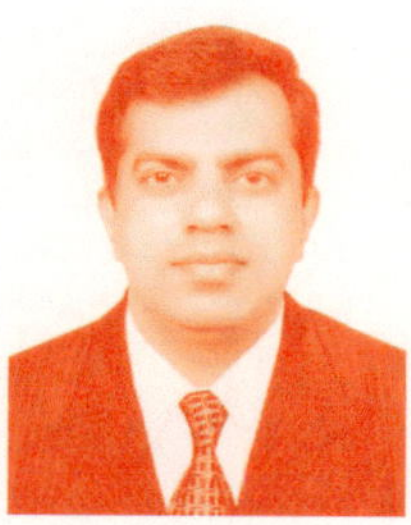
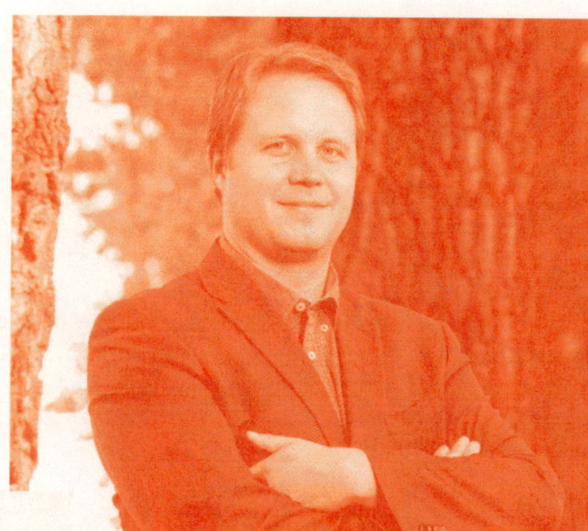
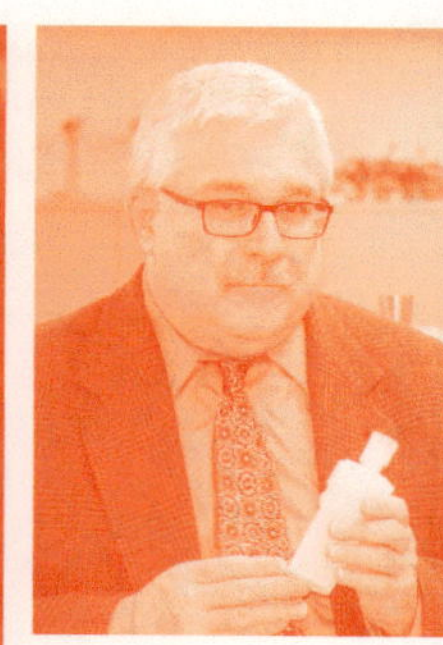
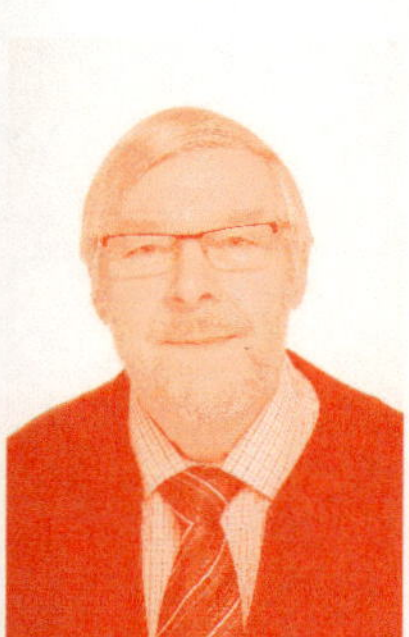
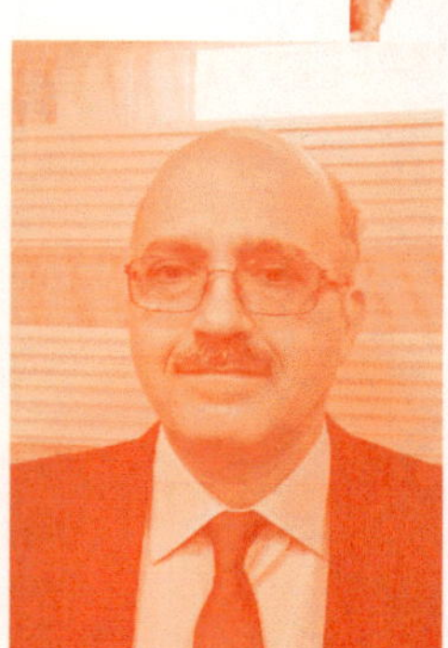
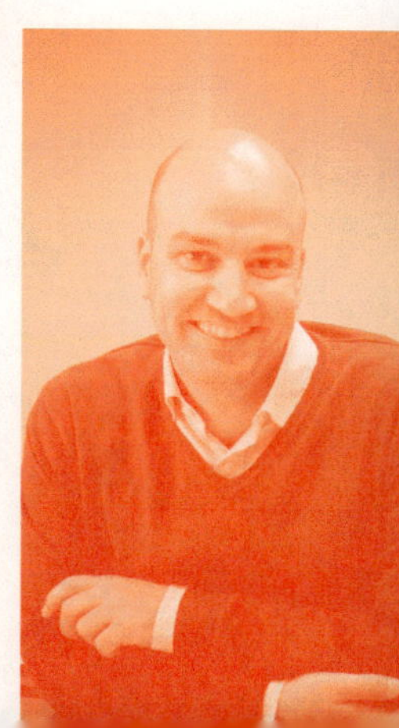
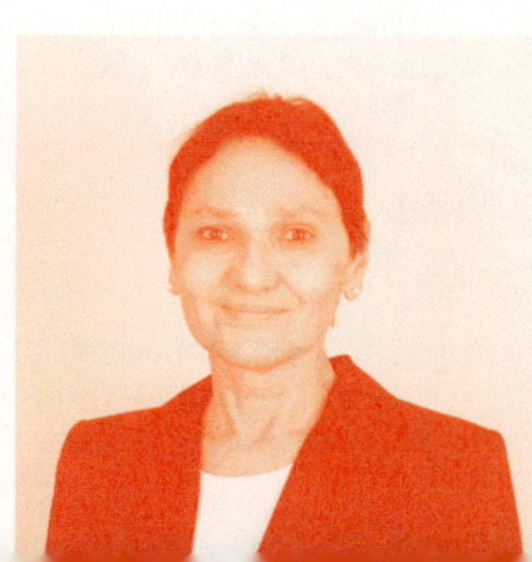

Fungal Infection
http://dx.doi.org/10.5772/intechopen.73887
Edited by Érico Silva de Loreto and Juliana Simoni Moraes Tondolo

Contributors
Jorge Cortes, Ivohne Corrales, Jacob Mensah-Attipoe, Oluyemi Olagoke Toyinbo, Monika Novak Babič, Jerneja Zupančič, Nina Gunde-Cimerman, Adolfo Paz Silva, Antonio Miguel Palomero Salinero, María Isabel Silva Torres, Mathilde Voinot Meissner, María Vilá Pena, Ángel Romasanta Blanco, José Pedreira García, Rita Sánchez-Andrade Fernández, José Ángel Hernández Malagón, Cristiana Cazapal-Monteiro, María Sol Arias Vázquez, Vira Lubenets, Viktoriya Havryliak, Nataliya Stadnytska, Diana Baranovych, Sofiya Vasylyuk, Olena Karpenko, Volodymyr Novikov, Michal Olszewski, Jintao Xu, Peter Wiliamson, Érico Silva de Loreto

First published in London, United Kingdom, 2019 by IntechOpen
IntechOpen is the global imprint of INTECHOPEN LIMITED, registered in England and Wales, registration number: 11086078, The Shard, 25th floor, 32 London Bridge Street
London, SE19SG – United Kingdom
Printed in Croatia

British Library Cataloguing-in-Publication Data
A catalogue record for this book is available from the British Library

Additional hard copies can be obtained from orders@intechopen.com

Fungal Infection
Edited by Érico Silva de Loreto and Juliana Simoni Moraes Tondolo
p. cm.
Print ISBN 978-1-83880-468-8
Online ISBN 978-1-83880-469-5
eBook (PDF) ISBN 978-1-83880-761-0

For EU product safety concerns:
IN TECH d.o.o., Prolaz Marije Krucifikse Kozulić 3, 51000 Rijeka, Croatia, info@intechopen.com or visit our website at intechopen.com.

Meet the editors

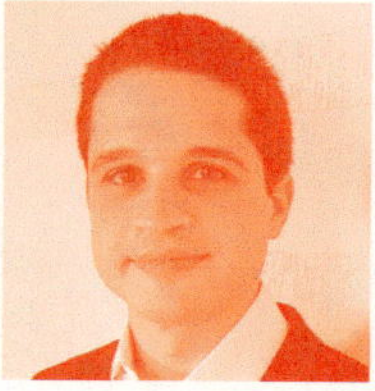

Dr. Érico Silva de Loreto is a professor at and a deputy director of the SOBRESP—Faculty of Health Sciences, Santa Maria, RS, Brazil. Prof. Dr. Loreto is a specialist in clinical laboratory and holds a master's and PhD in pharmaceutical sciences, a PhD in biological sciences (toxicological biochemistry), and a post-doctorate in pharmacology. His current research focus is on antimicrobial susceptibility testing, microbiological techniques for identification of microorganisms, pythiosis, and opportunistic fungal pathogens. His scientific production includes nearly 50 papers and a book chapter.

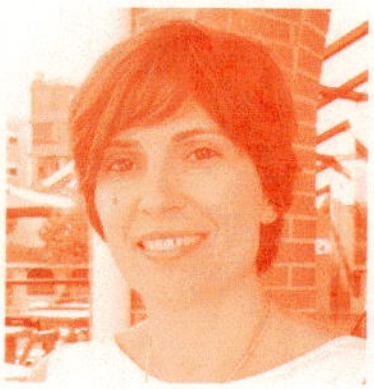

Professor Dr. Juliana Simoni Moraes Tondolo received her pharmaceutical degree and a master's and PhD in pharmacology from Federal University of Santa Maria. She also holds a master's in homeopathy and is a specialist in clinical laboratory. Throughout her career, she has worked as a homeopathic pharmacist and a biochemist at a military hospital; she has spent the last decade in full-time scientific research. Her main areas of interest have included antimicrobial susceptibility testing, pythiosis, and conidiobolomycosis, as well as immunology of fungal infections and extraction of fungal glucans with immunotherapeutic potential. She has written nearly 30 scientific papers and a book chapter, and she is currently a professor of psychopharmacology at SOBRESP—Faculty of Health Sciences.

Contents

Preface

A broad variety of fungi can cause fungal infections and lead to life-threatening diseases, typically in critically ill patients. Several risk factors are significantly associated with the development of invasive fungal infections, including immunosuppression, broad-spectrum antibiotics, total parenteral nutrition, mechanical ventilation, breakdown of anatomical barriers, and fungal colonization. Despite therapeutic advances in diagnostic techniques, prophylaxis, and treatment regimens, invasive fungal infections are still important causes of morbidity and mortality, and several groups of patients remain susceptible to these types of infections.

Fungi are heterotrophic organisms that can parasitize animals, plants, and even other fungi, using them as a source of nutrients. It is important to study these interactions in order to understand how these species adapt and cause infections in mammals. So, knowing how these microorganisms are distributed and how they respond to environmental pressures is critical for determining the epidemiology of the diseases they engender.

This book is organized in a collection of writings by experts from distinct research areas, aiming to provide up-to-date information on the epidemiology of fungal infections, host-pathogen interactions, the relationships between fungal growth and the environment, the use of fungal species to control soil parasites, and the antifungal properties of thiosulfonates.

On behalf of all the authors, I would like to warmly thank Ms. Sara Debeuc, from IntechOpen, who has tirelessly contributed to and assisted in the success of this publication.

Érico Silva de Loreto and Juliana Simoni Moraes Tondolo
SOBRESP—Faculty of Health Sciences,
Santa Maria, RS, Brazil

Section 1

Clinical Mycology

Chapter 1

Introductory Chapter: Epidemiology of Invasive Fungal Infection - An Overview

Erico S. Loreto and Juliana S.M. Tondolo

1. Introduction

Invasive fungal infections (IFIs) are a significant cause of morbidity and mortality in hospitalized patients and the immunocompromised populations. Candidemia, invasive aspergillosis, mucormycosis, cryptococcosis, and *Pneumocystis* pneumonia (PCP) are IFIs associated with the highest incidence and mortality. The broader use of more aggressive treatment modalities, such as hematopoietic stem cell transplantation (HSCT) and solid organ transplantation (SOT), as well as chemotherapy for cancer patients and prolonged corticosteroid therapy, has increased the population of immunocompromised patients at risk for IFIs. Other groups at risk include individuals who have HIV/AIDS in which PCP is an AIDS-defining disease [1]. In this chapter, we aim to overview the epidemiology of the leading causes of IFIs in humans.

2. Aspergillosis

The genus *Aspergillus* contains more than 300 species described and is divided into 20 sections [2]. However, only a few are known to cause human disease. Human aspergillosis is primarily caused by *Aspergillus fumigatus* (the most common species described in aspergillosis cases), *A. flavus*, *A. niger*, *A. terreus*, and *A. nidulans*. *Aspergillus* species are ubiquitous, are found in soil and several organic debris, and produce conidia that are easily aerosolized. These conidia, when inhaled, can colonize the host's lungs, which can develop various clinical syndromes depending on their degree of immunocompetence. Ingestion of spores via the gastrointestinal tract or direct inoculation via skin injuries is an uncommon way of inoculation [3–5].

The major risk factors for infection include prolonged neutropenia, HSCT, SOT, corticosteroid therapy, chronic granulomatous disease, immunosuppressive treatment for malignancies, hematologic malignancy, myelodysplastic syndrome or aplastic anemia, advanced stage of human immunodeficiency virus (HIV) infection (facilitated by low $CD4^+$ cell counts), previous infections (such as cytomegalovirus infection), and patients with critical illness [4, 6]. The spectrum of disease is determined by the host's immune status and the virulence of *Aspergillus* species.

In immunocompetent hosts, aspergillosis causes mainly allergic symptoms without invasion and destruction of the host's tissues and chronic pulmonary aspergillosis. Allergic bronchopulmonary aspergillosis (ABPA) is a syndrome that arises from a hypersensitivity reaction to antigens from *Aspergillus* and may be developed in patients with asthma and cystic fibrosis [7]. In the chronic pulmonary aspergillosis, a preexisting pulmonary condition is generally observed. Chronic cavitary

IntechOpen

pulmonary aspergillosis (aspergilloma or fungus ball) is the best-recognized form of pulmonary involvement due to *Aspergillus*, usually occurring in a preformed cavity in the lung (due to tuberculosis, sarcoidosis, or other necrotizing pulmonary processes) or in the paranasal sinuses [8, 9]. Subacute invasive aspergillosis (also called chronic necrotizing pulmonary aspergillosis) is a locally destructive invasion of lung parenchyma without invasion or dissemination to other organs [9, 10].

In immunocompromised patients, invasive aspergillosis (IA) can be a rapidly, progressive and frequently fatal disease. Invasive pulmonary aspergillosis (IPA) and rhinocerebral aspergillosis are the most common clinical forms of IA. Other clinical conditions included tracheobronchitis, invasive *Aspergillus* infection of the eye or heart, gastrointestinal invasive aspergillosis, cutaneous aspergillosis, and disseminated invasive aspergillosis [5]. Data from the Transplant-Associated Infection Surveillance Network (TRANSNET) [11] described that in HSCT recipients, invasive aspergillosis was the most common IFI (425 cases, 43%), followed by invasive candidiasis (276 cases, 28%) and zygomycosis (77 cases; 8%). One-year overall mortality rate reaches 75% [11]. In the Prospective Antifungal Therapy Alliance (PATH Alliance®) registry, from a cohort study of 960 cases of proven/probable IA, 48.3% of patients had hematologic malignancy, 29.2% received SOT, 27.9% were HSCT recipients, and 33.8% were neutropenic. The lung was the organ most frequently affected (76% of cases). The tracheobronchial tree, sinuses, skin, soft tissues, and the central nervous system were the most common extrapulmonary sites of infections. The most predominant species was *A. fumigatus* (72.6%), followed by *A. flavus* (9.9%), *A. niger* (8.7%), and *A. terreus* (4.3%). Overall Kaplan-Meier survival (12-week post-diagnosis) among all patients with IA was 64.4%.

3. Candidiasis

Candida species are ubiquitous yeasts, being frequent colonizers of the skin and normal flora of mucocutaneous membranes of humans. Also, it was also recovered from soil, hospital environment, food, inanimate objects, and nonanimal environments [12]. *Candida albicans*, *Candida dubliniensis*, *Candida glabrata*, *Candida guilliermondii*, *Candida intermedia*, *Candida kefyr*, *Candida krusei*, *Candida lusitaniae*, *Candida parapsilosis*, *Candida pseudotropicalis*, *Candida stellatoidea*, and *Candida tropicalis* are the main species associated with candidiasis, although more than 200 species of *Candida* have been identified.

Candida albicans remains the predominant species in most studies [13]. However, a shift in the etiology can be observed in different regions of the world [14]. For example, in northwestern Europe and the United States, *Candida glabrata* is generally recovered as the most common species, whereas in Southern Europe, some Asian countries and Latin America, *Candida parapsilosis* and *Candida tropicalis* are more frequently recovered than *Candida glabrata*. Of notable concern is the emergence of *Candida auris*, a multiresistant species associated with outbreaks of candidemia in many countries that presents a serious global health threat [12, 14–16].

As opportunistic pathogens, *Candida* infections can occur due to factors related to the host, the microorganism, or both. The three major conditions that predispose the human infection are: (i) the use of broad-spectrum antibiotics (long-term and/or repeated use), (ii) mucosal barrier breakdown, such as those induced by cytotoxic chemotherapy and medical interventions, and (iii) iatrogenic immunosuppression, such as corticosteroid therapy or chemotherapy-induced neutropenia [15]. Long hospital or intensive care unit (ICU) stay is the most common health care-associated risk [17]. Among the several virulence factors described for *Candida*, (i) the ability of most species to switch between yeast, pseudohypha, and hyphae morphotypes; (ii) the secretion of a variety of factors, such as secreted aspartyl proteases, phospholipases and candidalysin toxin; and (iii) the effective capacity of adherence (mediated by proteins such as agglutinin-like protein 3) and biofilm formation are the main microorganism-related factors that contribute to candidiasis [15].

The incidence of *Candida* infections varies according to several epidemiological and geographic characteristics. *Candida* species are among the top four main pathogens causing health care-associated bloodstream infections, particularly in ICU, affecting 250,000 people and causing more than 50,000 deaths worldwide every year, based on conservative estimates [18–20]. In an international study of prevalence and outcomes of infection in ICU, *Candida* was the third most common cause of infection (17%), after *Staphylococcus aureus* (20.5%) and *Pseudomonas* species (19.9%) [21].

Candida was the most common fungal pathogen that causes invasive infection in SOT population [22]. In bone marrow transplantation (BMT) under fluconazole prophylaxis, *Aspergillus* species replaced *Candida* as main cause of IFI [11]. Newborn infants [23], HIV-infected patient (without the use of antiretroviral therapy) [24], and patients who underwent abdominal surgery [25] are other populations at increased risk for *Candida* infections. Unadjusted mortality rates vary widely (from 29 to 76%) for candidemia. In the United States, the attributed mortality rate ranges from >30 to 40% and the median cost for inpatient care was $46,684 [15, 19, 26, 27].

4. Cryptococcosis

Cryptococcus neoformans and *Cryptococcus gattii* are the two species that commonly cause cryptococcosis in humans. Historically, these species were classified into three varieties, five serotypes, and eight molecular subtypes. However, based on phylogenetic and genotyping studies, it was proposed to split *Cryptococcus neoformans* into two species (*Cryptococcus deneoformans* and *Cryptococcus neoformans*) and *Cryptococcus gattii* into five species (*Cryptococcus bacillisporus*, *Cryptococcus decagatti*, *Cryptococcus deuterogattii*, *Cryptococcus gattii*, and *Cryptococcus tetragattii*) [28]. Nonetheless, considering that more data about the genetic diversity of *Cryptococcus* were recently described and the absence of defined biological and clinical differences between the seven new species, some authors recommend the use of "*Cryptococcus neoformans* species complex" and "*Cryptococcus gattii* species complex" as a practical intermediate step until this species differentiation is clinically relevant [29].

Cryptococcus neoformans has been isolated in decaying material within hollows of several tree species, fruit, and soil enriched by avian excreta (such as feral pigeons) and is globally distributed. *Cryptococcus gattii* is classically associated with eucalyptus tree and limited to tropical and subtropical regions. However, recent outbreaks in Canada, Northern Europe, and Northern USA suggest that the ecological range of this species may not be fully recognized. Both species can survive and replicate in environmental scavengers such as free-living amoebae and nematodes [30, 31]. The respiratory tract is the main portal of entry for the aerosolized infectious particles from the disrupted and contaminated environment (soil, tree, or bird droppings-enriched areas). Lung and the central nervous system (CNS) are the primary sites of infection, but eyes, prostate, and skin can be frequently involved. Traumatic inoculation may occur but is infrequent [31–33].

HIV infection, idiopathic CD4+ lymphopenia, corticosteroid treatment, SOT, malignant and lymphoproliferative disorders, sarcoidosis, treatment with some monoclonal antibodies (such as alemtuzumab, infliximab, etanercept, adalimumab, or anti-GM CSF), rheumatologic diseases (such as systemic lupus erythematosus and rheumatoid arthritis), chronic liver disease, renal failure and/or peritoneal dialysis, hyper-IgM syndrome or hyper-IgE syndrome are the main risk factors for cryptococcosis [31, 33, 34].

Cryptococcus infections in humans were considered uncommon before the 1970s. Cryptococcosis incidence increased significantly in the HIV epidemics in the 1980s. The overall incidence of 0.8 cases per million persons per year in the pre-AIDS era reached almost five cases per 100,000 persons per year in the peak of the AIDS epidemic. The incidence of cryptococcosis declined and stabilized from the mid-1990s with the use of fluconazole for the treatment of oral candidiasis and with the widespread use of active antiretroviral therapy (ART) [34–36]. However, HIV-associated cryptococcosis mortality remains unacceptably high, and globally, cryptococcal meningitis accounts for 15% of AIDS-related deaths. Cryptococcal infection-related deaths were estimated at 181,100 globally, with 75% (135,900) occurring in sub-Saharan Africa [37–39].

In HIV-negative individuals, cryptococcosis occurs in transplant recipients and other patients with primary or acquired defects in cell-mediated immunity [32]. In a recently multicenter, longitudinal cohort study in the United States [40], the demographics of 145 HIV-negative patients with cryptococcosis demonstrated that SOT (49 cases, 33.8%) was the main underlying disease, followed by autoimmune syndromes (15.9%), hematologic malignancy (11.7%), decompensated liver disease (9.7%), solid tumor (5.6%), primary immunodeficiency (2.1%), and HSCT (2.8%). Glucocorticoid therapy and cytotoxic chemotherapy were the immunosuppressive medications described for more than 40% of patients. CNS involvement was observed in 71 patients (49%).

5. Mucormycosis

Rhizopus is the most common genera causative of human disease, followed by *Mucor*, *Lichtheimia*, *Apophysomyces*, *Rhizomucor*, and *Cunninghamella* species. Less frequently, members include *Actinomucor*, *Cokeromyces*, *Saksenaea*, and *Syncephalastrum* [41–43]. These members from Mucorales family are ubiquitous in the environment, are taken by the host via inhalation of spores or ingestion of contaminated food, but rarely cause infection without obvious predisposing host factors [44].

Uncontrolled diabetes, hematological malignancy, malnutrition, solid organ transplantation, hematopoietic stem cell transplant, and liver disease are the primary underlying conditions associated with mucormycosis. Predisposing factors include corticosteroid use, neutropenia, trauma, anticancer therapy, use of calcineurin inhibitors, biological and renal replacement therapies, prior antifungal prophylaxis (e.g., voriconazole), iron overload and deferoxamine therapy [41, 42, 44].

Rhinocerebral, pulmonary, cutaneous, gastrointestinal, and disseminated mucormycosis are the common types of disease described. The mortality and morbidity rates are dependent on affected organ, Mucorales species, and medical status of the patient. Mucormycosis can be an extremely aggressive disease, and mortality rates can reach 46% in sinus infection, 73% in mucormycosis after exposure to voriconazole, 76% in pulmonary disease, and 96% in disseminated infections [42, 45].

Based on autopsy reports [46], mucormycosis is the third most common cause of invasive fungal infection, after candidiasis and aspergillosis. In developed countries, hematologic malignancies and hematopoietic stem cell transplantation are the leading underlying conditions in mucormycosis cases while in developing countries, particularly in India, the major causes of the disease are associated with uncontrolled diabetes or trauma [43, 47]. Data from Transplant-Associated Infection Surveillance Network show that mucormycosis (formerly zygomycosis) was the third most common IFI (8%) in HSCT [11] and sixth most common IFI (2%) among organ transplant recipients [22].

6. Pneumocystis

Pneumocystis jirovecii (previously *Pneumocystis carinii* f. sp. hominis) is an opportunistic pathogen causing pneumonia in patients with immunodeficiencies and can colonize the lung of healthy individuals. Initially classified as a protozoan species, it is now recognized as a fungus based on phylogenetic data and the genus comprising a group of highly diversified species with a high degree of hosts-species specificity [48]. The environmental reservoir was not identified so that the mammalian hosts can be considered as reservoirs. Indeed, it was demonstrated that close person-to-person contact could facilitate the transmission, and nosocomial transmission has been reported [48, 49].

Despite the genus *Pneumocystis* being known for years, its life cycle remains poorly understood, principally by the lack of a reliable continuous culture system. The hypothesized life cycle comprises different morphologic forms: trophozoites, cysts, and intracystic bodies (sporozoites) and all these forms reside in the alveoli of the lung with the cyst being considered the infectant and transmissible form [48, 50]. Evidence suggests that the gateway to infection is through inhalation since controlled studies in different animal models have demonstrated airborne transmission [48, 51]. As the organism is host specific, transmission from animals to humans is unlikely [51].

The occurrence of *Pneumocystis* pneumonia (PCP) is related to severely immunocompromised people, principally in HIV/AIDS patients, and with other immunosuppressed conditions, that is, cancers, autoimmune disorders, transplantation, chronic lung disease, especially obstructive pulmonary disease (COPD) [48]. Colonization rates have been reported on the order of 20–69% for HIV patients, from 0 to 20% for healthy adults, and in 6% of organ transplant recipients if no prophylaxis is given [51]. Primary exposure appears to occur at early childhood as demonstrated by the seroconversion seen in 85% of children up to 20 months of age [52]. Colonization of both children and adults may be a source of transmission of *Pneumocystis jirovecii*, serving as potential reservoirs. Guidelines for prevention and treatment of opportunistic infections in HIV-infected adults and adolescents include: treating patients with PCP together with prophylaxis of susceptible individuals (HIV patients with CD4 counts of <200 cells/μl or CD4 percentages of <14%); it is also recommended that a patient with PCP should not be placed in the same room with an immunodeficient patient. The prophylaxis among transplant recipients has been proved to be the most effective approach for ending outbreaks of PCP [48, 53].

7. Conclusions

The changes in the spectrum of the fungal infections associated with new risk factors and the emergence of resistant fungi highlight the necessity of a continuous update on knowledge of the epidemiology of fungal infections. Besides, the reduction of mortality among patients with IFIs must be accompanied by research that allows the development of new antifungal treatment strategies and earlier diagnosis by traditional and non-culture-based molecular tests.

Author details

Erico S. Loreto* and Juliana S. M. Tondolo
Sobresp Faculdade de Ciências da Saúde, RS, Brazil

*Address all correspondence to: erico.loreto@gmail.com

References

[1] Brown GD, Denning DW, Gow NA, Levitz SM, Netea MG, White TC. Hidden killers: Human fungal infections. Science Translational Medicine. 2012;**4**:165rv13. DOI: 10.1126/scitranslmed.3004404

[2] Samson RA, Visagie CM, Houbraken J, Hong SB, Hubka V, Klaassen CH, et al. Phylogeny, identification and nomenclature of the genus *Aspergillus*. Studies in Mycology. 2014;**78**:141-173. DOI: 10.1016/j.simyco.2014.07.004

[3] Dagenais TR, Keller NP. Pathogenesis of *Aspergillus fumigatus* in invasive aspergillosis. Clinical Microbiology Reviews. 2009;**22**:447-465. DOI: 10.1128/CMR.00055-08

[4] Challa S. Pathogenesis and pathology of invasive aspergillosis. Current Fungal Infection Reports. 2018;**12**:23-32. DOI: 10.1007/s12281-018-0310-4

[5] Bellmann-Weiler R, Bellmann R. Clinical Syndromes: *Aspergillus*. In: Presterl E, editor. Clinically Relevant Mycoses. 1st ed. New York, NY: Springer Berlin Heidelberg; 2019. pp. 77-89

[6] Patterson TF, Thompson GR 3rd, Denning DW, Fishman JA, Hadley S, Herbrecht R, et al. Practice guidelines for the diagnosis and management of aspergillosis: 2016 update by the Infectious Diseases Society of America. Clinical Infectious Diseases. 2016;**63**: e1-e60. DOI: 10.1093/cid/ciw326

[7] McCrary K. Allergic bronchopulmonary aspergillosis. In: Craig T, Ledford DK, editors. Allergy and Asthma. 1st ed. Switzerland, Cham: Springer; 2019. pp. 1-10

[8] Kim JS, So SS, Kwon SH. The increasing incidence of paranasal sinus fungus ball: A retrospective cohort study in two hundred forty-five patients for fifteen years. Clinical Otolaryngology. 2017;**42**:175-179. DOI: 10.1111/coa.12588

[9] Kanj A, Abdallah N, Soubani AO. The spectrum of pulmonary aspergillosis. Respiratory Medicine. 2018;**141**:121-131. DOI: 10.1016/j.rmed.2018.06.029

[10] Dogra V, Sinha AK, Saxena R, Talwar D. *Aspergillus* march: From ABPA to aspergilloma to subacute invasive aspergillosis. Allergy, Asthma and Clinical Immunology. 2016;**12**:64. DOI: 10.1186/s13223-016-0170-9

[11] Kontoyiannis DP, Marr KA, Park BJ, Alexander BD, Anaissie EJ, Walsh TJ, et al. Prospective surveillance for invasive fungal infections in hematopoietic stem cell transplant recipients, 2001-2006: Overview of the transplant-associated infection surveillance network (TRANSNET) database. Clinical Infectious Diseases. 2010;**50**:1091-1100. DOI: 10.1086/651263

[12] Ruhnke M. Clinical syndromes: *Candida* and Candidosis. In: Presterl E, editor. Clinically Relevant Mycoses. 1st ed. New York, NY: Springer Berlin Heidelberg; 2019. pp. 45-75

[13] Dadar M, Tiwari R, Karthik K, Chakraborty S, Shahali Y, Dhama K. *Candida albicans* - Biology, molecular characterization, pathogenicity, and advances in diagnosis and control - An update. Microbial Pathogenesis. 2018;**117**:128-138. DOI: 10.1016/j.micpath.2018.02.028

[14] Quindos G, Marcos-Arias C, San-Millan R, Mateo E, Eraso E. The continuous changes in the aetiology and epidemiology of invasive candidiasis: From familiar *Candida albicans* to multiresistant *Candida auris*. International Microbiology. 2018;**21**:107-119. DOI: 10.1007/s10123-018-0014-1

[15] Pappas PG, Lionakis MS, Arendrup MC, Ostrosky-Zeichner L, Kullberg BJ. Invasive candidiasis. Nature Reviews. Disease Primers. 2018;**4**:18026. DOI: 10.1038/nrdp.2018.26

[16] Lockhart SR, Etienne KA, Vallabhaneni S, Farooqi J, Chowdhary A, Govender NP, et al. Simultaneous emergence of multidrug-resistant *Candida auris* on 3 continents confirmed by whole-genome sequencing and epidemiological analyses. Clinical Infectious Diseases. 2017;**64**:134-140. DOI: 10.1093/cid/ciw691

[17] Pfaller MA, Diekema DJ. Epidemiology of invasive candidiasis: A persistent public health problem. Clinical Microbiology Reviews. 2007; **20**:133-163. DOI: 10.1128/CMR. 00029-06

[18] Kullberg BJ, Arendrup MC. Invasive candidiasis. The New England Journal of Medicine. 2015;**373**:1445-1456. DOI: 10.1056/NEJMra1315399

[19] Wisplinghoff H, Bischoff T, Tallent SM, Seifert H, Wenzel RP, Edmond MB. Nosocomial bloodstream infections in US hospitals: Analysis of 24,179 cases from a prospective nationwide surveillance study. Clinical Infectious Diseases. 2004;**39**:309-317. DOI: 10.1086/421946

[20] Magill SS, Edwards JR, Bamberg W, Beldavs ZG, Dumyati G, Kainer MA, et al. Multistate point-prevalence survey of health care-associated infections. The New England Journal of Medicine. 2014;**370**:1198-1208. DOI: 10.1056/NEJMoa1306801

[21] Vincent JL, Rello J, Marshall J, Silva E, Anzueto A, Martin CD, et al. International study of the prevalence and outcomes of infection in intensive care units. Journal of the American Medical Association. 2009;**302**:2323-2329. DOI: 10.1001/jama.2009.1754

[22] Pappas PG, Alexander BD, Andes DR, Hadley S, Kauffman CA, Freifeld A, et al. Invasive fungal infections among organ transplant recipients: Results of the transplant-associated infection surveillance network (TRANSNET). Clinical Infectious Diseases. 2010;**50**:1101-1111. DOI: 10.1086/651262

[23] Shetty SS, Harrison LH, Hajjeh RA, Taylor T, Mirza SA, Schmidt AB, et al. Determining risk factors for candidemia among newborn infants from population-based surveillance: Baltimore, Maryland, 1998-2000. Pediatric Infectious Disease Journal. 2005;**24**:601-604

[24] Auclair S, Liu F, Hu H. Loss of immune control in HIV-infected patients: How does mucosal candidiasis occur? Future Microbiology. 2017;**12**: 5-8. DOI: 10.2217/fmb-2016-0194

[25] Bassetti M, Righi E, Ansaldi F, Merelli M, Scarparo C, Antonelli M, et al. A multicenter multinational study of abdominal candidiasis: Epidemiology, outcomes and predictors of mortality. Intensive Care Medicine. 2015;**41**:1601-1610. DOI: 10.1007/s00134-015-3866-2

[26] Strollo S, Lionakis MS, Adjemian J, Steiner CA, Prevots DR. Epidemiology of hospitalizations associated with invasive candidiasis, United States, 2002-2012. Emerging Infectious Diseases. 2017;**23**:7-13. DOI: 10.3201/eid2301.161198

[27] Cleveland AA, Farley MM, Harrison LH, Stein B, Hollick R, Lockhart SR, et al. Changes in incidence and antifungal drug resistance in candidemia: Results from population-based laboratory surveillance in Atlanta and Baltimore, 2008-2011. Clinical Infectious Diseases. 2012;**55**:1352-1361. DOI: 10.1093/cid/cis697

[28] Hagen F, Khayhan K, Theelen B, Kolecka A, Polacheck I, Sionov E,

et al. Recognition of seven species in the *Cryptococcus gattii*/*Cryptococcus neoformans* species complex. Fungal Genetics and Biology. 2015;**78**:16-48. DOI: 10.1016/j.fgb.2015.02.009

[29] Kwon-Chung KJ, Bennett JE, Wickes BL, Meyer W, Cuomo CA, Wollenburg KR, et al. The case for adopting the "species complex" nomenclature for the etiologic agents of cryptococcosis. mSphere. 2017;**2**:e00357-e00316. DOI: 10.1128/mSphere.00357-16

[30] May RC, Stone NR, Wiesner DL, Bicanic T, Nielsen K. *Cryptococcus*: From environmental saprophyte to global pathogen. Nature Reviews Microbiology. 2016;**14**:106-117. DOI: 10.1038/nrmicro.2015.6

[31] Maziarz EK, Perfect JR. Cryptococcosis. Infectious Disease Clinics of North America. 2016;**30**: 179-206. DOI: 10.1016/j.idc.2015.10.006

[32] Williamson PR, Jarvis JN, Panackal AA, Fisher MC, Molloy SF, Loyse A, et al. Cryptococcal meningitis: Epidemiology, immunology, diagnosis and therapy. Nature Reviews Neurology. 2017;**13**:13-24. DOI: 10.1038/nrneurol.2016.167

[33] Guery R, Lanternier F, Lortholary O. Clinical Syndromes: Cryptococcosis. In: Presterl E, editor. Clinically Relevant Mycoses. 1st ed. New York, NY: Springer Berlin Heidelberg; 2019. pp. 101-111

[34] Perfect JR. Cryptococcosis (*Cryptococcus neoformans* and *Cryptococcus gattii*). In: Bennett JE, Dolin R, Blaser MJ, editors. Mandell, Douglas, and Bennett's principles and practice of infectious diseases. 8th ed. Philadelphia, PA: Elsevier/Saunders; 2015. pp. 2934-2948

[35] Hajjeh RA, Conn LA, Stephens DS, Baughman W, Hamill R, Graviss E, et al. Cryptococcosis: Population-based multistate active surveillance and risk factors in human immunodeficiency virus-infected persons. Cryptococcal Active Surveillance Group. The Journal of Infectious Diseases. 1999;**179**: 449-454. DOI: 10.1086/314606

[36] van Elden LJ, Walenkamp AM, Lipovsky MM, Reiss P, Meis JF, de Marie S, et al. Declining number of patients with cryptococcosis in the Netherlands in the era of highly active antiretroviral therapy. AIDS. 2000;**14**:2787-2788

[37] Pasquier E, Kunda J, De Beaudrap P, Loyse A, Temfack E, Molloy SF, et al. Long-term mortality and disability in cryptococcal meningitis: A systematic literature review. Clinical Infectious Diseases. 2018;**66**:1122-1132. DOI: 10.1093/cid/cix870

[38] Goldberg DW, Tenforde MW, Mitchell HK, Jarvis JN. Neurological sequelae of adult meningitis in Africa: A systematic literature review. Open Forum Infectious Diseases. 2018;**5**:ofx246. DOI: 10.1093/ofid/ofx246

[39] Rajasingham R, Smith RM, Park BJ, Jarvis JN, Govender NP, Chiller TM, et al. Global burden of disease of HIV-associated cryptococcal meningitis: An updated analysis. The Lancet Infectious Diseases. 2017;**17**:873-881. DOI: 10.1016/S1473-3099(17)30243-8

[40] Marr KA, Sun Y, Spec A, Lu N, Panackal A, Bennett J, et al. A multicenter, longitudinal cohort study of cryptococcosis in HIV-negative people in the United States. Clinical Infectious Diseases. 2019. DOI: 10.1093/cid/ciz193

[41] Jeong W, Keighley C, Wolfe R, Lee WL, Slavin MA, Kong DCM, et al. The epidemiology and clinical manifestations of mucormycosis: A systematic review and meta-analysis of case reports. Clinical Microbiology and Infection. 2019;**25**:26-34. DOI: 10.1016/j.cmi.2018.07.011

[42] Roden MM, Zaoutis TE, Buchanan WL, Knudsen TA, Sarkisova TA, Schaufele RL, et al. Epidemiology and outcome of zygomycosis: A review of 929 reported cases. Clinical Infectious Diseases. 2005;**41**:634-653. DOI: 10.1086/432579

[43] Challa S. Mucormycosis: Pathogenesis and pathology. Current Fungal Infection Reports. 2019;**54**: S16-S22. DOI: 10.1007/s12281-019-0337-1

[44] Hassan MIA, Voigt K. Pathogenicity patterns of mucormycosis: Epidemiology, interaction with immune cells and virulence factors. Medical Mycology. 2019;**57**:S245-S256. DOI: 10.1093/mmy/myz011

[45] Trifilio SM, Bennett CL, Yarnold PR, McKoy JM, Parada J, Mehta J, et al. Breakthrough zygomycosis after voriconazole administration among patients with hematologic malignancies who receive hematopoietic stem-cell transplants or intensive chemotherapy. Bone Marrow Transplantation. 2007;**39**:425-429. DOI: 10.1038/sj.bmt.1705614

[46] Dignani MC. Epidemiology of invasive fungal diseases on the basis of autopsy reports. F1000Prime Reports. 2014;**6**:81. DOI: 10.12703/P6-81

[47] Petrikkos G, Skiada A, Lortholary O, Roilides E, Walsh TJ, Kontoyiannis DP. Epidemiology and clinical manifestations of mucormycosis. Clinical Infectious Diseases. 2012;**54**(Suppl 1):S23-S34. DOI: 10.1093/cid/cir866

[48] Ma L, Cisse OH, Kovacs JA. A molecular window into the biology and epidemiology of Pneumocystis spp. Clinical Microbiology Reviews. 2018;**31**:e00009-18. DOI: 10.1128/CMR.00009-18

[49] Gianella S, Haeberli L, Joos B, Ledergerber B, Wuthrich RP, Weber R, et al. Molecular evidence of interhuman transmission in an outbreak of *Pneumocystis jirovecii* pneumonia among renal transplant recipients. Transplant Infectious Disease. 2010;**12**:1-10. DOI: 10.1111/j.1399-3062.2009.00447.x

[50] Cushion MT, Linke MJ, Ashbaugh A, Sesterhenn T, Collins MS, Lynch K, et al. Echinocandin treatment of pneumocystis pneumonia in rodent models depletes cysts leaving trophic burdens that cannot transmit the infection. PLoS One. 2010;**5**:e8524. DOI: 10.1371/journal.pone.0008524

[51] Morris A, Norris KA. Colonization by *Pneumocystis jirovecii* and its role in disease. Clinical Microbiology Reviews. 2012;**25**:297-317. DOI: 10.1128/CMR.00013-12

[52] Vargas SL, Hughes WT, Santolaya ME, Ulloa AV, Ponce CA, Cabrera CE, et al. Search for primary infection by *Pneumocystis carinii* in a cohort of normal, healthy infants. Clinical Infectious Diseases. 2001;**32**:855-861

[53] de Boer MG, Kroon FP, le Cessie S, de Fijter JW, van Dissel JT. Risk factors for *Pneumocystis jirovecii* pneumonia in kidney transplant recipients and appraisal of strategies for selective use of chemoprophylaxis. Transplant Infectious Disease. 2011;**13**:559-569. DOI: 10.1111/j.1399-3062.2011.00645.x

Chapter 2

Cryptococcus neoformans-Host Interactions Determine Disease Outcomes

Jintao Xu, Peter R. Wiliamson and Michal A. Olszewski

Abstract

The fungal pathogen *Cryptococcus neoformans* can infect the central nervous system (CNS) and cause fatal meningoencephalitis, which accounts for an estimated 180,000 deaths per year. Cryptococcal meningoencephalitis (CM) occurs mainly in the individuals with compromised immune systems. Thus, cryptococcal disease in the CNS has been predominantly attributed to insufficient immune responses and subsequent uncontrolled fungal growth. However, evidence has emerged that an inappropriate immune response, as much as an insufficient response, may promote clinical deterioration and pathogenesis. In this chapter, we will review the different types of immune responses to *C. neoformans* and their contribution to tissue damage and diseases.

Keywords: *Cryptococcus neoformans*, pathogenesis, immune pathology

1. Introduction

The human fungal pathogen *Cryptococcus neoformans* causes substantial morbidity and mortality worldwide, with an estimated 1 million infections and 180,000 deaths per year [1–3]. Although the primary route of infection is through inhalation of yeast into the lungs, fungal dissemination to the central nervous system (CNS) leads to severe meningoencephalitis that can cause death or long-lasting neurological sequelae, including memory loss, vision deficiencies, hearing and speech impairments, and motor deficits [4–6]. Treatment options for cryptococcal meningoencephalitis (CM) are limited and often unsuccessful due to the increasing development of drug resistance, the high toxicity of the antifungal drugs and the poor permeability of the blood brain barrier [7–9]. Unsuccessful treatments are often accompanied with high mortality rates up to 15% and relapse rates of 30–50% [10–12]. Thus, there is a pressing need for understanding the pathogenesis of *C. neoformans* infection to develop more effective therapeutic strategies.

Cryptococcal infections usually manifest in patients who are immunocompromised secondary to HIV infection, cancer therapies, or organ transplantation [3]. This has led to the characterization of *C. neoformans* as an "opportunistic pathogen" that causes disease only when the immune system cannot control its growth. Prior studies have established a central role for T cell mediated immunity in fungal clearance from the lungs and suggested that T-cell mediated immunity is also beneficial in the CNS [13–25]. These studies also support a paradigm that clinical failures are predominantly due to a deficiency in microbiological control. However, attempts to develop immunotherapies that enhance the immune responses in CM have been largely unsuccessful, indicating other factors may also participate in the disease pathology [26]. Furthermore, clinical and experimental studies increasingly show that an exaggerated host immune response can promote cryptococcal pathogenesis. For example, a common complication of CM in HIV/AIDS patients is the immune reconstitution inflammatory syndrome (cIRIS) that develops after initiation of anti-retroviral therapy [27, 28]. A parallel syndrome occurs among non-HIV patients with severe cryptococcal CNS infection, termed post infectious immune inflammatory syndrome (PIIRS) [29–31]. These patients develop severe neurological sequela and morbidity with persisting inflammatory responses, often despite fungal eradication [28, 32–36]. A detrimental role of host inflammation is further supported by the therapeutic effects of corticosteroids in ameliorating IRIS and PIIRS symptoms and by observations that premature or abrupt steroid-weaning may result in the recurrence of CNS lesions and clinical relapse [29, 30, 37].

This evidence challenges the view that cryptococcal disease is a consequence of a compromised immune system. Instead, the outcomes of cryptococcal disease can be better understood as a balance of *C. neoformans*-host interactions. The effect of *C. neoformans* on host disease can be explained by the damage-response framework (DRF), a theory for microbial pathogenesis proposed in 1999 [38]. The DRF theory incorporates the contributions of host-microbe interaction, rather than presenting microbial pathogenesis as a singular outcome of either microbial factors or host factors. The results of host-microbe interaction can be visualized with a single parabola depicting host damage as a function of the strength of the immune response [26]. Weak host immune responses due to HIV infection or immunosuppressive therapies fail to control fungal growth, which results in fungus-mediated host damage. However, strong immune responses elicited by *C. neoformans* can also lead to host damages and diseases. In this chapter, we will review recent human clinical and experimental animal studies that have enhanced our understanding of the complex mechanisms involved in immunopathogenesis during *C. neoformans* infection. Uncovering the mechanisms that are involved in anticryptococcal host defense or in immunopathogenesis will facilitate the discovery of new intervention strategies to treat cryptococcal infections.

2. Cryptococcal immune reconstitution inflammatory syndrome

C. neoformans can cause infection in both the meninges and the Virchow-Robin channels surrounding the penetrating vessels within the brain parenchyma [39]. Although the exact mechanism by which this encapsulated pathogen migrates into the CNS is currently unclear, studies have found that circulating *C. neoformans* was trapped in the brain capillary and can actively transmigrate the microvasculature with contributions from urease and metalloprotease [40–42]. After migration, *C. neoformans* causes fatal meningoencephalitis which accounts for 15–20% of AIDS-related deaths [1, 43, 44]. The high fungal burdens during CM in AIDS are associated with mortality, suggesting a prominent role of the fungal pathogen for host damage [45]. Thus, in HIV infection/AIDS, susceptibility to CM is thought to occur due to lack of T cell-mediated fungal clearance. Indeed, studies have shown that presence of CSF cytokine and chemokine responses consisting primarily of IL-6, IFN-γ, IL-8, IL-10, IL-17, CCL5 and TNF-α, are associated with increased macrophage activation, more rapid fungal clearance from the CSF, and patient survival [45]. The overall low levels of cytokine production in AIDS patients and insufficient activation of resident or recruited macrophages in the absence of T cells producing IFN-γ/TNF-α lead to uncontrolled fungal growth [45, 46].

Antiretroviral therapy (ART) in AIDS patients rapidly restores host T cell responses. However, in a portion of patients it leads to a highly lethal complication, cIRIS, which is defined as a paradoxical clinical deterioration after initiation of ART, despite efficient control of fungal infection [28]. cIRIS occurs in 15–30% of HIV-infected individuals with cryptococcosis [28, 47]. Similarly, patients who undergo immune suppressive regiments during bone marrow transplantation or autoimmune diseases can develop cIRIS like syndromes once the host immune response is restored when immunosuppressive therapy is tapered [48]. Previous studies have found that paucity of initial CSF inflammation, low IFN-γ levels, and high fungal loads are risk factors for the development of IRIS [27, 45]. During cIRIS, the immune response in the brain is characterized by excessive activation of Th1 CD4+ subsets with elevated production of cytokines including IFN-γ and TNF-α [27, 33, 49].

While the exact pathogenic mechanisms of IRIS have not been unraveled, the lymphopenic environment during HIV infection may result in abnormal function of residual CD4 T cells, rendering them more pathogenic as the population expands after ART [50]. Furthermore, it has also been proposed that there exists a decoupling of innate and adaptive immune responses in AIDS patients prior to ART due to deficient T cell responses, which sets the stage for excessive inflammation after T cell reconstitution. Indeed, several lines of evidence show that mononuclear immune cells are implicated in cIRIS. Predisposition to cIRIS has been shown to be associated with higher CCL2/MCP-1, CCL3/MIP-1α, and GMCSF production in the CSF, which promotes trafficking and activation of macrophages in the infection sites [45]. Patients with cIRIS had increased numbers of proinflammatory intermediate monocytes (CD14highCD16+) which produce reactive oxygen species [51, 52]. Although macrophages can be primed by fungal pathogens in AIDS patients prior to ART, they never become fully activated in the absence of T cell help to exert their effector functions in fungal clearance. This results in high levels of pathogen replication as the disease progresses. Nevertheless, increasing numbers of primed macrophages accumulate and create a state of immunological hyperresponsiveness to the subsequently CD4+ T cell help. ART rapidly restores Th1 type response in the host with high level of IFN-γ production. Large numbers of primed macrophages then become fully activated to produce an acute spike in proinflammatory mediators, which may drive immunopathology during cIRIS. Thus, macrophage activation in cIRIS may act in concert with T-cell responses resulting in tissue-destructive inflammatory responses.

The mechanisms of tissue damage by host inflammation during fungal infections are still under active research. Macrophage or T cell production of TNF-α, IL-1β, reactive oxygen species (ROS) and nitrogen species (RNS), may contribute to irreversible tissue damage and/or lead to neuronal apoptosis [53–55]. *C. neoformans* infection also induces cerebral edema and raised CSF pressure that are associated with symptoms including headache, nausea, and mental status deterioration.

3. Postinfectious inflammatory response syndrome

Another example showing that strong host immune responses during *C. neoformans* infection can induce immunopathology is post-infectious inflammatory response syndrome (PIIRS). It is characterized in non-HIV patients during initial therapy by severe mental deficits despite antifungal therapy and their apparent immunocompetent state. Reports showed that up to 25% of cases in the United States and 60% in the Far East occur in apparently immune competent patients [56, 57]. Despite antifungal therapy and negative CSF-*C. neoformans* cultures, PIIRS patients many times require ventricle-peritoneal shunts to relieve the high CSF pressure caused by inflammation. Recent studies have shown that patients with PIIRS exhibit strong intrathecal Th1 responses with high levels of IFN-γ production and a relatively lack of Th2 responses [30]. Importantly, elevated levels of CSF neurofilament light chain (NFL), a marker of axonal injury, indicate ongoing immunological host neuron damage. Interestingly, macrophages recruited to the CNS infection site are often alternatively activated (M2) and exhibit poor phagocytic effect during PIIRS [30]. This apparent Th1-M2 discrepancy suggests that PIIRS patients may have downstream defects in monocyte activation. New therapies that consider immune-mediated host injury may decrease mortality in these severe or refractory clinical cases [43].

4. Animal models of IRIS and PIIRS

Detrimental roles for immune responses in the pathogenesis of cryptococcus-associated IRIS or PIIRS have also been recently demonstrated in experimental mouse models. A recent study in our lab established a reproducible mouse model of CM using C57BL/6 mice infected intravenously with 10^6 CFU of *C. neoformans* strain 52D [58]. Using this model, we found that infected mice displayed overt and severe symptoms similar to that of human patients, including increased cranial pressure, ataxia, and limb paralysis after 21 days post infection (dpi). Importantly, over 50% of animals succumbed to infection between 21 and 35 dpi, despite apparent fungal control in the CNS (**Figure 1**). Thus, we showed that the magnitude of CNS fungal burden does not directly correlate with the intensity of disease symptoms or mortality during CM.

Brain cellular inflammation, marked by leukocyte accumulation after 21 dpi and dominated by CD4+ T cell infiltration, plays an important role in the pathology of the CNS in cryptococcal-infected mice. Similar to human patients with IRIS and PIIRS, infiltrating CD4+ T cells in brains of cryptococcal-infected mice exhibit a Th1-type bias and produce high levels of IFN-γ. Critically, the influx of immune cells into the CNS after 21 dpi was synchronized with the onset of fungal clearance, development of neurological symptoms, and mortality. The depletion of CD4 + T cells leads to a reduction in mortality and inflammatory pathology, providing conceptual evidence that CD4 + T cells are a principal mediator of inflammation and pathology in this model. Notably, over the course of the study, the survival of CD4+

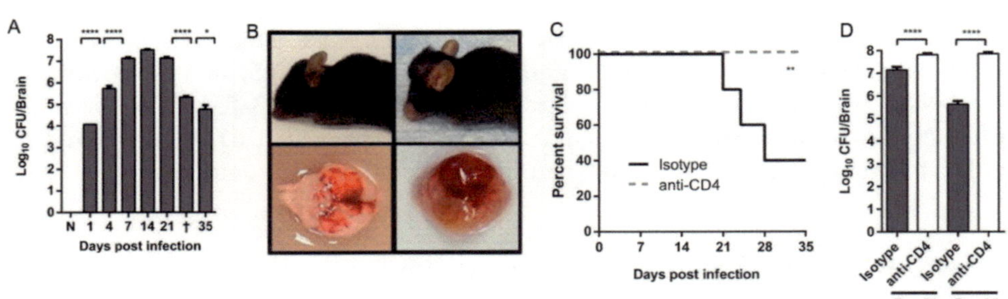

Figure 1.
*Depletion of CD4+ T cells resulted in improved survival despite higher fungal burden during CM. C57BL/6 mice were infected with 10^6 CFU of C. neoformans 52D via retro-orbital intravenous inoculation. (A) Fungal burdens were measured in whole-brain homogenates at the indicated time points. Naive mice and animals that succumbed to infection (†) are indicated. (B) Representative images of severe cranial swelling and CNS tissue injury in infected mice. (C) Survival of infected CD4-depleted (broken line) and isotype-treated mice through 35 dpi. (D) Brain fungal burdens were calculated on day 21 and 35 dpi. *, $P < 0.05$; **, $P < 0.01$; ****, $P < 0.0001$. Reproduced from Neal et al., [58].*

T cell depleted mice significantly improved despite having higher fungal loads in the CNS compared to mice with sufficient CD4+ T cells (**Figure 1**). Depletion of CD4+ T cells during CM also broadly inhibited all other aspects of the CNS inflammatory response, including accumulation of CD8+ T cells and CD11b + Ly6C+ myeloid effector cells. Taken together, these data strongly support the idea that CD4+ T cells exert dual but opposing roles during CM: promoting the elimination of the fungal pathogen in the CNS but simultaneously driving tissue damage, neurological deterioration, and death.

Another animal model has also demonstrated the pathological role of CD4+ T cells in cIRIS. Eschke and colleagues reconstituted RAG$^{-/-}$ mice, which are deficient in T and B cells, with WT CD4+ T cells after infection with *C. neoformans* [59]. They found that mice receiving CD4 T cells displayed high levels of Th1-type cytokines such as TNF-α and IFN-γ compared to mice not receiving CD4+ T cells. These results suggested that CD4+ T cell reconstitution in mice infected with *C. neoformans* may lead to syndromes similar to IRIS in HIV-infected patients [59]. These animal models provide important tools for further investigating the mechanism of cryptococcal pathology.

5. Host immunity to *C. neoformans* infection: protective or non-protective, the yin and yang

Protective immunity is conferred by a fine balance between immune responses that eliminate the pathogen and those that limit host damages. However, an immune response induced by the pathogen may be non-protective for any one or combination of the following reasons: (1) it could occur in the wrong location or timeframe, promoting inflammatory injury without effective clearance of pathogens; (2) it could be too strong and cause immunopathology despite control of pathogen burden; 3) regulatory mechanisms meant to maintain host tissue integrity may lead to microbial survival and persistence and thus result in chronic inflammation. Below, we describe cellular and molecular mechanisms by which dysregulation of immune responses contribute to host disease during infection with *C. neoformans*.

5.1 Host immune responses contribute to fungal clearance but also tissue damage

Upon infection, *C. neoformans* is sensed by a variety of innate receptors including Toll-like receptors [60–62], mannose receptors [60], and β-glucan receptors [63–65]. Macrophages [66, 67], DCs [68], natural killer cells [69–72] and neutrophils [73] have been shown to mediate killing *C. neoformans*, however, the development of the adaptive immune response is required for controlling the fungal growth in the host [74–76]. Specifically, the development of Th1 and Th17 responses that are associated with classical activation of macrophages (M1) promotes fungal clearance in both humans and experimental mouse models [14, 77]. DCs and macrophages function as the potential sensors for infection through PRRs or inflammasomes, and produce cytokines such as IL-12, IL-23, IL-6, IL-18, TNF-α and IL-1β, which have been shown to promote the Th1/Th17 response during *C. neoformans* infection [78–84]. During this response, Th1 and Th17 cells produce cytokines such as IFN-γ, IL-17 and IL-22, which act on macrophages, neutrophils or epithelial cells and induce robust antimicrobial and phagocytic responses, including the production of reactive oxygen and nitrogen species [16, 85–90]. As a result, resident and/or recruited macrophages and DCs can become highly activated and function as the main effector cells for controlling fungal infection [91, 92].

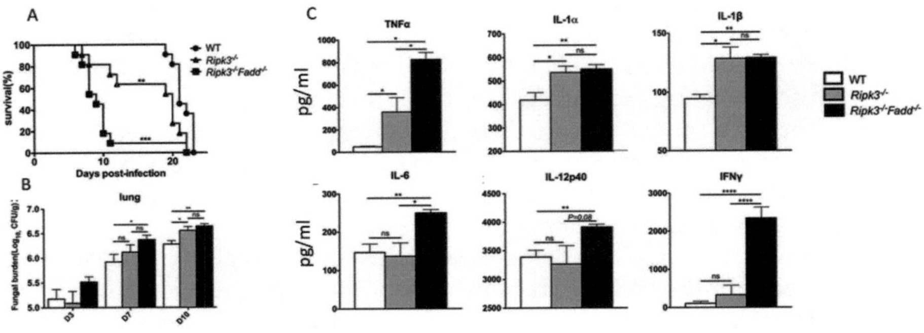

Figure 2.
*RIPK3 and FADD modulate host responses against C. neoformans infection. (A) Ripk3$^{-/-}$ and Ripk3$^{-/-}$Fadd$^{-/-}$ mice were more susceptible to C. neoformans infection. (B) Diminished fungal clearance in lungs of Ripk3$^{-/-}$ and Ripk3$^{-/-}$Fadd$^{-/-}$ mice. (C) RIPK3 or FADD deletions altered Th-polarizing and pro-inflammatory cytokine profiles in pulmonary response to cryptococcal infection. *, $P < 0.05$; **, $P < 0.01$; ****, $P < 0.0001$. Reproduced from Fa et al., [93].*

Although generation of the Th1/Th17 response and subsequent M1 activation play a critical role in controlling fungal growth, excessive immune responses can become destructive and cause lung immunopathology following fungal infection. Recent studies demonstrated that FADD and RIPK3 proteins, which are mediators of death receptor-triggered extrinsic apoptosis, play a crucial immune regulatory role in preventing excessive inflammation during *C. neoformans* infection [93]. Deletion of RIPK3 and FADD led to a robust Th1-biased response with M1-biased macrophage activation, which is accompanied by marked upregulation of cytokines like TNF-α, IL-1α, IL-1β, IL6, and IFN-γ (**Figure 2**). Rather than being protective, this robust host response was deleterious and is associated with paradoxical fungal growth and rapid clinical deterioration (**Figure 2**). These findings showed that excessive inflammation can mediate tissue damage and host disease during cryptococcal infection [93]. Furthermore, the balance between Th1 and Th17 immune responses plays important roles in optimizing clearance and minimizing inflammatory damage to the host tissues during fungal infections. For example, it has been shown that IL-23 and Th17 pathway act as a negative regulator of Th1 response and thus contribute to fungal growth during *C. albicans* and *A. fumigatus* infection [94]. Recent studies show that the Th1, Th2, Th17 responses and cytokines co-exist and evolve during different time points in a chronic fungal infection [13], while fungus adapts to and exploit the dysregulation of this immune balance. Thus, therapeutic cytokines and vaccines may create a new therapeutic mean to restore protective host responses and fungal control, but would need to be introduced with extreme caution not to induce an excessive immune bias.

DCs play a critical role in modulating host antifungal responses. Distinct PRRs and intracellular signaling pathways in DCs help to define the immune response to fungal pathogens [95]. Studies from Bonifazi *et al.* showed that *C. albicans* exploits multiple, functionally distinct, receptor-signaling pathways in DCs ultimately affecting the local inflammatory/anti-inflammatory state in the gut [96]. Furthermore, depletion of DC through administration of diphtheria toxin to transgenic mice resulted in rapid clinical deterioration and death of mice infected with *C. neoformans* [97]. Early mortality in DC-depleted mice was related to increased neutrophil accumulation accompanied with histopathologic evidence of alveolar damage, including hemorrhagic and proteinaceous exudates [97]. Similar changes mediated by neutrophils were associated with respiratory failure and death [98]. Collectively, these data define an important role for DC in regulating the initial innate and adaptive response following fungal infections.

5.2 Host immune responses normally associated with homeostasis can contribute to fungal persistence

Cryptococcal virulence includes evasion of immune recognition, interference with phagocytosis, and modulation of host immune responses [56, 99]. Many fungal factors have been shown to promote allergic Th2 or Treg responses. These types of responses are characterized by alternatively activated macrophages and may promote uncontrolled fungal growth [56]. However, the regulatory immune response is also crucial for maintaining host tissue homeostasis and limiting the inflammatory responses that can cause tissue damage.

Th2: In murine models, *C. neoformans* exhibits a remarkable ability to induce Th2 response, which is associated with fungal growth, fungus-associated allergic responses and disease relapse. Although rare for *C. neoformans* infection, other fungal pathogens such as *Aspergillus fumigatus* can induce devastating allergic bronchopulmonary mycosis in human patients that is accompanied by a Th2 response [100, 101]. Additionally, enhancing the Th2 response in a mouse model has been shown to exacerbate pulmonary disease during cryptococcal infection, supporting a causal role of Th2 response in pathology [102].

IL-4 and IL-13 provide the most potent proximal signals for Th2 cell polarization [13, 17, 103]. The epithelial-derived cytokines thymic stromal lymphopoietin (TSLP), IL-25, and IL-33 have been shown to regulate the development of Th2 response during asthma [104, 105]. A time-dependent increase in IL-33 expression in the lungs has been found during *C. neoformans* infection, and IL-33 signaling can promote Th2 response and facilitates cryptococcal growth in the lungs [106]. In addition, chitin recognition via host chitotriosidase promotes harmful Th2 cell differentiation by CD11b + conventional DCs in response to pulmonary fungal infection [102]. However, Th2 polarization may play beneficial roles at certain stage of infection. IL-4Ra has been shown to afford protection early upon infection associated with increased IFN-γ and nitric oxide production. More importantly, Th2 response plays important roles in wound healing to tissue destructive pathogens [107] and down regulating inflammatory responses [108]. Many of the proteins produced in response to IL-4 and IL-13, such as arginase, MMP12, and TREM-2, are associated with injury [109]. Th2-activated macrophages also produce TGF-β which can suppress pro-inflammatory responses while at the same time serving as a potent pro-fibrotic mediator [110].

Treg: CD4+ CD25+ Treg cells expressing the transcription factor forkhead box protein 3 (FoxP3) play critical roles in down-regulating immune responses and promoting homeostasis [111, 112]. Accumulation of antigen specific Treg has been shown during infection with fungal pathogens [113–116]. Multiple studies have shown that Treg can suppress effector cells and lead to fungal persistence. For example, Treg in mice infected with *C. albicans* were shown to be capable of inhibiting Th1 activity, thereby limiting protective responses. However, the roles of Treg in modulating Th17 activity are still controversial, with both positive and negative effects reported [117, 118]. Similar enhancement of effector function in the absence of Treg can be found in multiple other models of viral, bacterial, and parasitic infection [119].

While Treg may lead to pathogen persistence, they can actually be beneficial in protecting against immune-mediated damage to the host. This has been demonstrated in diseases caused by *Pneumocystis pneumonia*, HSV, *Schistosoma mansoni* where depletion of Treg leads to enhanced pathology [120–123]. It has been shown that depletion of Tregs enhanced Th2 response during pulmonary cryptococcal infection as evidenced by increased mucus production, enhanced eosinophilia, and increased IgE production [113]. Interestingly, Treg-depleted mice exhibited elevated fungal burden compared to control mice, suggesting that Treg mediated enhanced fungal control by inhibiting non-protective Th2 responses [113]. Confirming these observations, therapeutic expansion of Tregs during pulmonary cryptococcal infection has been shown to limit allergic airway inflammation, as demonstrated by reduced production of IgE and Th2 cytokines [116, 124]. Since laboratory mice show a strong tendency to develop a detrimental Th2 response during *C. neoformans* infection, Tregs may be protective in this context by inhibiting the tissue-damaging Th2 response. Furthermore, Tregs have also been demonstrated to be required for resistance to reinfection with *C. albicans* [120].

IL-10 is a critical effector molecule involved in the immunoregulatory functions of Treg cells [125]. IL-10 has been reported to inhibit production of cytokines such as IL-1, IL-6, IL-23, IFN-γ, TNF-α and chemokines including CCL2(MCP-1), CCL12(MCP-5), CCL5(RANTES), IL-8, CXCL10(IP-10), and CXCL2(MIP-2) [126]. During *C. neoformans* infection, IL-10-deficient mice display reduced expression of IL-4, IL-5, and IL-13, but enhanced TNF-α and IL-12 expression [127]. Studies have further shown that IL-10 signaling blockade can promote fungal control even if administered after persistent infection has been established [128]. IL-10 expression also occurs and dampens fungal control in response to other fungal pathogens such as *C. albicans*, *H. capsulatum* and *A. fumigatus* [129–131]. These studies suggest that IL-10 production plays an essential role in the development of persistent fungal infections. Deficiency or blockade of IL-10 may result in better fungal control, however, it comes at the cost of excessive inflammation that may cause greater tissue damage [127, 132, 133].

The roles of Tregs in the CNS during fungal infection, however, remain less studied. One report shows an increase in the abundance of Treg cells within cIRIS patients [134]. Further clinical and animal studies are needed to investigate the functions of Tregs during fungal CNS infections.

6. Conclusions and future directions

A tightly-regulated balance between inflammatory and regulatory mechanisms is required to control fungal infection, maintain host homeostasis, and ultimately develop protective immunity (**Figure 3**). Recent studies have demonstrated that disease and mortality in cryptococcal infection can result from either uncontrolled fungal growth due to defective host immunity, or excessive host inflammation. As the spectrum of hosts with cryptococcal disease expands, it is critical to understand and distinguish pathology caused by the pathogen or host responses. For example, additional suppression of weak immunity by steroid therapy in patients with uncontrolled fungal growth may lead to enhanced fungus-mediated damage and mortality in HIV-associated cryptococcal patients [135]. Instead, adjunctive IFN-γ therapy to bolstering immunity in these patients has the potential to ameliorate fungus-mediated damage and mortality [136]. However, in cIRIS patients, who experience inflammation-mediated tissue damage and mortality, corticosteroids can be effective to control disease-related deterioration [30]. Furthermore, mounting evidence implies that the top priority for cIRIS and PIIRS is to control the devastating immunopathology. Thus, comprehensive therapeutic strategies that take fungus- and host mediated damage into account could have the potential to significantly improve therapeutic outcomes.

Recent studies have identified the involvement of a number of immunopathogenic mechanisms including CD4+ T cells. However, the function of CD4 T cells overlaps with the mechanisms required for fungal clearance. Little is known about whether it is possible to uncouple the anti-fungal host defense mechanisms from the host immune responses that mediate deleterious immunopathology. One of

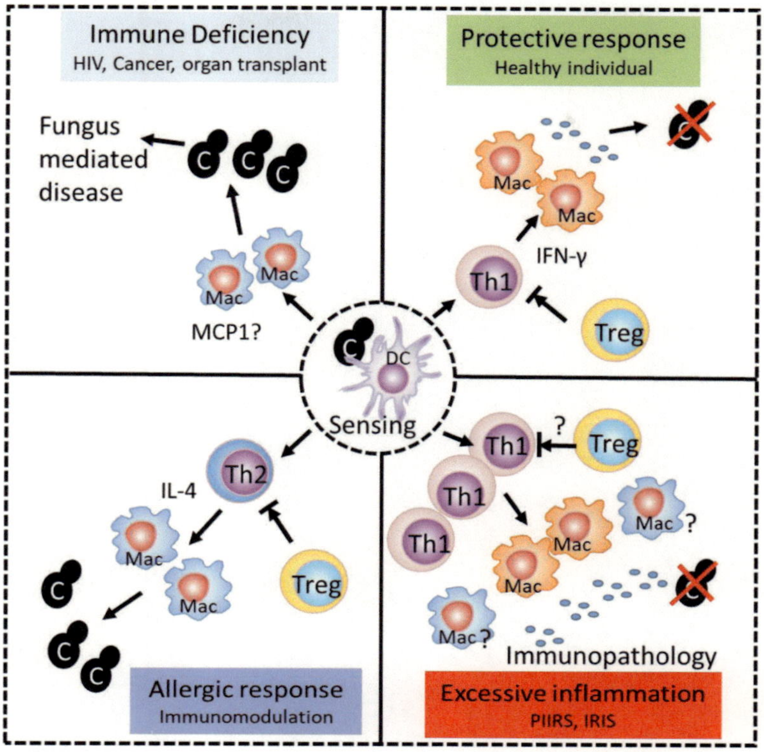

Figure 3.
C. neoformans and host interactions determine disease outcomes. In the center, innate immune cells such as DCs recognize C. neoformans using multiple pattern recognition receptors. A weak immune response due to HIV, cancer, or organ transplant can result in fungal-mediated tissue damage. Macrophages recruited into the infected tissue without T cell stimulation fail to control fungal growth. In healthy individuals, the DC-initiated Th1 response, which completely activated macrophages to efficiently control C. neoformans infection. Cytokines such as TNF-α and IFN-γ, as well as iNOS, are critical for fungal control. Tregs play important roles in limiting inflammation and maintaining homeostasis of the host. During IRIS and PIIRS, however, excessive inflammation can cause tissue damage despite fungal control. Whether Tregs are functional under this state is not clear. Macrophages may not be activated in PIIRS patients even with strong Th1 and IFN-γ production. Overproduction of cytokines and iNOS may promote tissue damage and cause disease. For certain host genetic backgrounds or highly virulent strains, an allergic Th2 response is developed and control of fungal growth fails. Host tissue damage in this circumstance may stem from both the pathogen and the detrimental Th2 responses.

the future directions in this research field is to identify mechanisms that are not required for fungal clearance but are major culprits in immunopathology which could be promising targets for future immunotherapies.

Acknowledgements

The authors thank Mr. Mack Reynolds for thoughtful edit of the manuscript.

This work was supported in part by the Intramural Research Program of the NIH, NIAID, AI001123-01 and AI001124-01 to PRW and Veterans Administration Merit Review Awards to M.A.O. (1I01BX000656) and VA RCS Award M.A.O. (1IK6BX003615).

Conflict of interest

The authors declare that there is no conflict of interest regarding the publication of this article.

Author details

Jintao Xu[1,2*], Peter R. Wiliamson[3] and Michal A. Olszewski[1,2]

1 Division of Pulmonary and Critical Care Medicine, Department of Internal Medicine, University of Michigan Health System, Ann Arbor, Michigan, USA

2 Research Service, Ann Arbor VA Health System, Department of Veterans Affairs Health System, Ann Arbor, Michigan, USA

3 Laboratory of Clinical Immunology and Microbiology, National Institute of Allergy and Infectious Diseases (NIAID), National Institutes of Health (NIH), Bethesda, Maryland, USA

*Address all correspondence to: xxjjtt07@gmail.com

References

[1] Park BJ, Wannemuehler KA, Marston BJ, Govender N, Pappas PG, Chiller TM. Estimation of the current global burden of cryptococcal meningitis among persons living with HIV/AIDS. AIDS. 2009;**23**:525-530

[2] Pappas PG. Cryptococcal infections in non-HIV-infected patients. Transactions of the American Clinical and Climatological Association. 2013;**124**:61

[3] Rajasingham R, Smith RM, Park BJ, Jarvis JN, Govender NP, Chiller TM, et al. Global burden of disease of HIV-associated cryptococcal meningitis: An updated analysis. The Lancet Infectious Diseases. 2017;**17**:873-881

[4] González-Duarte A, Calleja JH, Mitre VG, Ramos GG. Simultaneous central nervous system complications of *C. neoformans* infection. Neurology International. 2009;**1**:e22

[5] Goldberg DW, Tenforde MW, Mitchell HK, Jarvis JN. Neurological sequelae of adult meningitis in Africa: A systematic literature review. In: Open Forum Infectious Diseases. USA: Oxford University Press; 2017. p. ofx246

[6] Beardsley J, Wolbers M, Kibengo FM, Ggayi A-BM, Kamali A, Cuc NTK, et al. Adjunctive dexamethasone in HIV-associated cryptococcal meningitis. New England Journal of Medicine. 2016;**374**:542-554

[7] Bicanic T, Harrison T, Niepieklo A, Dyakopu N, Meintjes G. Symptomatic relapse of HIV-associated cryptococcal meningitis after initial fluconazole monotherapy: The role of fluconazole resistance and immune reconstitution. Clinical Infectious Diseases. 2006;**43**:1069-1070

[8] Saag MS, Graybill RJ, Larsen RA, Pappas PG, Perfect JR, Powderly WG, et al. Practice guidelines for the management of cryptococcal disease. Clinical Infectious Diseases. 2000;**30**:710-718

[9] Perfect JR, Dismukes WE, Dromer F, Goldman DL, Graybill JR, Hamill RJ, et al. Clinical practice guidelines for the management of cryptococcal disease: 2010 update by the Infectious Diseases Society of America. Clinical Infectious Diseases. 2010;**50**:291-322

[10] Pappas PG, Perfect JR, Cloud GA, Larsen RA, Pankey GA, Lancaster DJ, et al. Cryptococcosis in human immunodeficiency virus-negative patients in the era of effective azole therapy. Clinical Infectious Diseases. 2001;**33**:690-699

[11] Lee Y-C, Wang J-T, Sun H-Y, Chen Y-C. Comparisons of clinical features and mortality of cryptococcal meningitis between patients with and without human immunodeficiency virus infection. Journal of Microbiology, Immunology and Infection. 2011;**44**: 338-345

[12] Musubire AK, Boulware DR, Meya DB, Rhein J. Diagnosis and management of cryptococcal relapse. Journal of AIDS & Clinical Research. 2013;Suppl **3**(3). pii: S3-003

[13] Arora S, Olszewski MA, Tsang TM, McDonald RA, Toews GB, Huffnagle GB. Effect of cytokine interplay on macrophage polarization during chronic pulmonary infection with *Cryptococcus neoformans*. Infection and Immunity. 2011;**79**(5):1915-1926

[14] Chen G-h, McNamara DA, Hernandez Y, Huffnagle GB, Toews GB, Olszewski MA. Inheritance of immune polarization patterns is linked to resistance versus susceptibility to *Cryptococcus neoformans* in a mouse model. Infection and Immunity. 2008;**76**:2379-2391

[15] Jain AV, Zhang Y, Fields WB, McNamara DA, Choe MY, Chen G-h, et al. Th2 but not Th1 immune bias results in altered lung functions in a murine model of pulmonary *Cryptococcus neoformans* infection. Infection and Immunity. 2009;77:5389-5399

[16] Murdock BJ, Huffnagle GB, Olszewski MA, Osterholzer JJ. Interleukin-17A enhances host defense against cryptococcal lung infection through effects mediated by leukocyte recruitment, activation, and gamma interferon production. Infection and Immunity. 2014;**82**:937-948

[17] Zhang Y, Wang F, Tompkins KC, McNamara A, Jain AV, Moore BB, et al. Robust Th1 and Th17 immunity supports pulmonary clearance but cannot prevent systemic dissemination of highly virulent *Cryptococcus neoformans* H99. The American Journal of Pathology. 2009;**175**:2489-2500

[18] Hardison SE, Ravi S, Wozniak KL, Young ML, Olszewski MA, Wormley FL Jr. Pulmonary infection with an interferon-γ-producing *Cryptococcus neoformans* strain results in classical macrophage activation and protection. The American Journal of Pathology. 2010;**176**:774-785

[19] Wozniak KL, Ravi S, Macias S, Young ML, Olszewski MA, Steele C, et al. Insights into the mechanisms of protective immunity against *Cryptococcus neoformans* infection using a mouse model of pulmonary cryptococcosis. PLoS One. 2009;**4**:e6854

[20] Wozniak KL, Young ML, Wormley FL. Protective immunity against experimental pulmonary cryptococcosis in T cell depleted mice. Clinical and Vaccine Immunology. 2011;**18**(5):717-723

[21] Huffnagle GB, McNeil LK. Dissemination of *C. neoformans* to the central nervous system: Role of chemokines, Th1 immunity and leukocyte recruitment. Journal of Neurovirology. 1999;**5**:76-81

[22] Uicker WC, McCracken JP, Buchanan KL. Role of CD4+ T cells in a protective immune response against *Cryptococcus neoformans* in the central nervous system. Sabouraudia. 2006;**44**:1-11

[23] Aguirre K, Crowe J, Haas A, Smith J. Resistance to *Cryptococcus neoformans* infection in the absence of CD4+ T cells. Medical Mycology. 2004;**42**:15-25

[24] Uicker WC, Doyle HA, McCracken JP, Langlois M, Buchanan KL. Cytokine and chemokine expression in the central nervous system associated with protective cell-mediated immunity against *Cryptococcus neoformans*. Medical Mycology. 2005;**43**:27-38

[25] Buchanan KL, Doyle HA. Requirement for CD4+ T lymphocytes in host resistance against *Cryptococcus neoformans* in the central nervous system of immunized mice. Infection and Immunity. 2000;**68**:456-462

[26] Pirofski L-a, Casadevall A. Immune-mediated damage completes the parabola: *Cryptococcus neoformans* pathogenesis can reflect the outcome of a weak or strong immune response. MBio. 2017;**8**:e02063-e02017

[27] Boulware DR, Bonham SC, Meya DB, Wiesner DL, Park GS, Kambugu A, et al. Paucity of initial cerebrospinal fluid inflammation in cryptococcal meningitis is associated with subsequent immune reconstitution inflammatory syndrome. The Journal of Infectious Diseases. 2010;**202**:962-970

[28] Haddow LJ, Colebunders R, Meintjes G, Lawn SD, Elliott JH, Manabe YC, et al. Cryptococcal immune reconstitution inflammatory syndrome in HIV-1-infected individuals: Proposed

clinical case definitions. The Lancet Infectious Diseases. 2010;**10**:791-802

[29] Panackal AA, Komori M, Kosa P, Khan O, Hammoud DA, Rosen LB, et al. Spinal arachnoiditis as a complication of cryptococcal meningoencephalitis in non-HIV previously healthy adults. Clinical Infectious Diseases. 2017;**64**:275-283

[30] Panackal AA, Wuest SC, Lin YC, Wu T, Zhang N, Kosa P, et al. Paradoxical immune responses in non-HIV cryptococcal meningitis. PLoS Pathogens. 2015;**11**:e1004884

[31] Williamson PR. Post-infectious inflammatory response syndrome (PIIRS): Dissociation of T-cell-macrophage signaling in previously healthy individuals with cryptococcal fungal meningoencephalitis. Macrophage (Houst). 2015;**2**:pii: e1078

[32] Barber DL, Andrade BB, Sereti I, Sher A. Immune reconstitution inflammatory syndrome: The trouble with immunity when you had none. Nature Reviews. Microbiology. 2012;**10**:150-156

[33] Boulware DR, Meya DB, Bergemann TL, Wiesner DL, Rhein J, Musubire A, et al. Clinical features and serum biomarkers in HIV immune reconstitution inflammatory syndrome after cryptococcal meningitis: A prospective cohort study. PLoS Medicine. 2010;**7**:e1000384

[34] Chang CC, Omarjee S, Lim A, Spelman T, Gosnell BI, Carr WH, et al. Chemokine levels and chemokine receptor expression in the blood and the cerebrospinal fluid of HIV-infected patients with cryptococcal meningitis and cryptococcosis-associated immune reconstitution inflammatory syndrome. The Journal of Infectious Diseases. 2013;**208**:1604-1612

[35] Meya DB, Manabe YC, Boulware DR, Janoff EN. The immunopathogenesis of cryptococcal immune reconstitution inflammatory syndrome: Understanding a conundrum. Current Opinion in Infectious Diseases. 2016;**29**:10-22

[36] Meya DB, Okurut S, Zziwa G, Rolfes MA, Kelsey M, Cose S, et al. Cellular immune activation in cerebrospinal fluid from ugandans with cryptococcal meningitis and immune reconstitution inflammatory syndrome. The Journal of Infectious Diseases. 2015;**211**:1597-1606

[37] Panackal AA, Marr KA, Williamson PR. Dexamethasone in cryptococcal meningitis. The New England Journal of Medicine. 2016;**375**:188

[38] Casadevall A, Pirofski L-a. Host-pathogen interactions: Redefining the basic concepts of virulence and pathogenicity. Infection and Immunity. 1999;**67**:3703-3713

[39] Lee SC, Dickson DW, Casadevall A. Pathology of cryptococcal meningoencephalitis: Analysis of 27 patients with pathogenetic implications. Human Pathology. 1996;**27**:839-847

[40] Shi M, Li SS, Zheng C, Jones GJ, Kim KS, Zhou H, et al. Real-time imaging of trapping and urease-dependent transmigration of *Cryptococcus neoformans* in mouse brain. The Journal of Clinical Investigation. 2010;**120**:1683-1693

[41] Vu K, Tham R, Uhrig JP, Thompson GR, Pombejra SN, Jamklang M, et al. Invasion of the central nervous system by *Cryptococcus neoformans* requires a secreted fungal metalloprotease. MBio. 2014;**5**:e01101-e01114

[42] Olszewski MA, Noverr MC, Chen G-H, Toews GB, Cox GM, Perfect JR, et al. Urease expression by *Cryptococcus neoformans* promotes microvascular sequestration, thereby enhancing central nervous system invasion.

The American Journal of Pathology. 2004;**164**:1761-1771

[43] Bratton EW, El Husseini N, Chastain CA, Lee MS, Poole C, Stürmer T, et al. Comparison and temporal trends of three groups with cryptococcosis: HIV-infected, solid organ transplant, and HIV-negative/non-transplant. PLoS One. 2012;**7**:e43582

[44] Brizendine KD, Baddley JW, Pappas PG. Predictors of mortality and differences in clinical features among patients with Cryptococcosis according to immune status. PLoS One. 2013;**8**:e60431

[45] Jarvis JN, Meintjes G, Bicanic T, Buffa V, Hogan L, Mo S, et al. Cerebrospinal fluid cytokine profiles predict risk of early mortality and immune reconstitution inflammatory syndrome in HIV-associated cryptococcal meningitis. PLoS Pathogens. 2015;**11**:e1004754

[46] Jarvis JN, Casazza JP, Stone HH, Meintjes G, Lawn SD, Levitz SM, et al. The phenotype of the Cryptococcus-specific CD4+ memory T-cell response is associated with disease severity and outcome in HIV-associated cryptococcal meningitis. The Journal of Infectious Diseases. 2013;**207**:1817-1828

[47] Williamson PR, Jarvis JN, Panackal AA, Fisher MC, Molloy SF, Loyse A, et al. Cryptococcal meningitis: Epidemiology, immunology, diagnosis and therapy. Nature Reviews Neurology. 2017;**13**:13

[48] Sun H-Y, Alexander BD, Huprikar S, Forrest GN, Bruno D, Lyon GM, et al. Predictors of immune reconstitution syndrome in organ transplant recipients with cryptococcosis: Implications for the management of immunosuppression. Clinical Infectious Diseases. 2014;**60**:36-44

[49] Worsley CM, Suchard MS, Stevens WS, Van Rie A, Murdoch DM. Multi-analyte profiling of ten cytokines in South African HIV-infected patients with immune reconstitution inflammatory syndrome (IRIS). AIDS Research and Therapy. 2010;**7**:36

[50] Krupica T Jr, Fry TJ, Mackall CL. Autoimmunity during lymphopenia: A two-hit model. Clinical Immunology. 2006;**120**:121-128

[51] Meya DB, Okurut S, Zziwa G, Rolfes MA, Kelsey M, Cose S, et al. Cellular immune activation in cerebrospinal fluid from Ugandans with cryptococcal meningitis and immune reconstitution inflammatory syndrome. The Journal of Infectious Diseases. 2014;**211**:1597-1606

[52] Scriven JE, Rhein J, Hullsiek KH, Von Hohenberg M, Linder G, Rolfes MA, et al. Early ART after cryptococcal meningitis is associated with cerebrospinal fluid pleocytosis and macrophage activation in a multisite randomized trial. The Journal of Infectious Diseases. 2015;**212**:769-778

[53] Lucchinetti C, Brück W, Parisi J, Scheithauer B, Rodriguez M, Lassmann H. Heterogeneity of multiple sclerosis lesions: Implications for the pathogenesis of demyelination. Annals of Neurology: Official Journal of the American Neurological Association and the Child Neurology Society. 2000;**47**:707-717

[54] Hendriks JJ, Teunissen CE, de Vries HE, Dijkstra CD. Macrophages and neurodegeneration. Brain Research Reviews. 2005;**48**:185-195

[55] Nikić I, Merkler D, Sorbara C, Brinkoetter M, Kreutzfeldt M, Bareyre FM, et al. A reversible form of axon damage in experimental autoimmune encephalomyelitis and multiple sclerosis. Nature Medicine. 2011;**17**:495

[56] Olszewski MA, Zhang Y, Huffnagle GB. Mechanisms of cryptococcal virulence and persistence. Future Microbiology. 2010;**5**:1269-1288

[57] Fang W, Fa Z, Liao W. Epidemiology of Cryptococcus and cryptococcosis in China. Fungal Genetics and Biology. 2015;**78**:7-15

[58] Neal LM, Xing E, Xu J, Kolbe JL, Osterholzer JJ, Segal BM, et al. CD4+ T cells orchestrate lethal immune pathology despite fungal clearance during *Cryptococcus neoformans* meningoencephalitis. MBio. 2017;**8**:e01415-e01417

[59] Eschke M, Piehler D, Schulze B, Richter T, Grahnert A, Protschka M, et al. A novel experimental model of *Cryptococcus neoformans*-related immune reconstitution inflammatory syndrome (IRIS) provides insights into pathogenesis. European Journal of Immunology. 2015;**45**:3339-3350

[60] Dan JM, Wang JP, Lee CK, Levitz SM. Cooperative stimulation of dendritic cells by *Cryptococcus neoformans* mannoproteins and CpG oligodeoxynucleotides. PLoS One. 2008;**3**:e2046

[61] Nakamura K, Miyazato A, Xiao G, Hatta M, Inden K, Aoyagi T, et al. Deoxynucleic acids from *Cryptococcus neoformans* activate myeloid dendritic cells via a TLR9-dependent pathway. The Journal of Immunology. 2008;**180**:4067-4074

[62] Biondo C, Midiri A, Messina L, Tomasello F, Garufi G, Catania MR, et al. MyD88 and TLR2, but not TLR4, are required for host defense against *Cryptococcus neoformans*. European Journal of Immunology. 2005;**35**:870-878

[63] Nakamura K, Kinjo T, Saijo S, Miyazato A, Adachi Y, Ohno N, et al. Dectin-1 is not required for the host defense to *Cryptococcus neoformans*. Microbiology and Immunology. 2007;**51**:1115-1119

[64] Campuzano A, Castro-Lopez N, Wozniak KL, Wager CML, Wormley FL Jr. Dectin-3 is not required for protection against *Cryptococcus neoformans* infection. PLoS One. 2017;**12**:e0169347

[65] Cross C, Bancroft G. Ingestion of acapsular *Cryptococcus neoformans* occurs via mannose and beta-glucan receptors, resulting in cytokine production and increased phagocytosis of the encapsulated form. Infection and Immunity. 1995;**63**:2604-2611

[66] Vecchiarelli A, Pietrella D, Dottorini M, Monari C, Retini C, Todisco T, et al. Encapsulation of *Cryptococcus neoformans* regulates fungicidal activity and the antigen presentation process in human alveolar macrophages. Clinical & Experimental Immunology. 1994;**98**:217-223

[67] Liu L, Tewari RP, Williamson PR. Laccase protects *Cryptococcus neoformans* from antifungal activity of alveolar macrophages. Infection and Immunity. 1999;**67**:6034-6039

[68] Wozniak KL, Levitz SM. *Cryptococcus neoformans* enters the endolysosomal pathway of dendritic cells and is killed by lysosomal components. Infection and Immunity. 2008;**76**:4764-4771

[69] Kawakami K, Koguchi Y, Qureshi MH, Yara S, Kinjo Y, Uezu K, et al. NK cells eliminate *Cryptococcus neoformans* by potentiating the fungicidal activity of macrophages rather than by directly killing them upon stimulation with IL-12 and IL-18. Microbiology and Immunology. 2000;**44**:1043-1050

[70] Wiseman JC, Ma LL, Marr KJ, Jones GJ, Mody CH. Perforin-dependent cryptococcal microbicidal activity in NK cells requires PI3K-dependent ERK1/2 signaling. The Journal of Immunology. 2007;**178**:6456-6464

[71] Xiang RF, Li S, Ogbomo H, Stack D, Mody CH. β1 Integrins are required to

mediate NK cell killing of *Cryptococcus neoformans*. The Journal of Immunology. 2018;**201**:2369-2376

[72] Li SS, Mody CH. NKp46 is an NK cell fungicidal pattern recognition receptor. Trends in Microbiology. 2016;**24**:929-931

[73] Chaturvedi V, Wong B, Newman SL. Oxidative killing of *Cryptococcus neoformans* by human neutrophils. Evidence that fungal mannitol protects by scavenging reactive oxygen intermediates. The Journal of Immunology. 1996;**156**:3836-3840

[74] Mody C, Lipscomb M, Street N, Toews G. Depletion of CD4+ (L3T4+) lymphocytes in vivo impairs murine host defense to *Cryptococcus neoformans*. The Journal of Immunology. 1990;**144**:1472-1477

[75] Lim T, Murphy J. Transfer of immunity to cryptococcosis by T-enriched splenic lymphocytes from *Cryptococcus neoformans*-sensitized mice. Infection and Immunity. 1980;**30**:5-11

[76] Mody CH, Paine R, Jackson C, Chen G-H, Toews GB. CD8 cells play a critical role in delayed type hypersensitivity to intact *Cryptococcus neoformans*. The Journal of Immunology. 1994;**152**:3970-3979

[77] Romani L. Immunity to fungal infections. Nature Reviews Immunology. 2011;**11**:275

[78] Kleinschek MA, Muller U, Brodie SJ, Stenzel W, Kohler G, Blumenschein WM, et al. IL-23 enhances the inflammatory cell response in *Cryptococcus neoformans* infection and induces a cytokine pattern distinct from IL-12. The Journal of Immunology. 2006;**176**:1098-1106

[79] Kawakami K, Tohyama M, Xie Q, Saito A. IL-12 protects mice against pulmonary and disseminated infection caused by *Cryptococcus neoformans*. Clinical & Experimental Immunology. 1996;**104**:208-214

[80] Kawakami K, Qureshi MH, Zhang T, Okamura H, Kurimoto M, Saito A. IL-18 protects mice against pulmonary and disseminated infection with *Cryptococcus neoformans* by inducing IFN-gamma production. The Journal of Immunology. 1997;**159**:5528-5534

[81] Siddiqui AA, Shattock RJ, Harrison TS. Role of capsule and interleukin-6 in long-term immune control of *Cryptococcus neoformans* infection by specifically activated human peripheral blood mononuclear cells. Infection and Immunity. 2006;**74**:5302-5310

[82] Huffnagle GB, Toews GB, Burdick MD, Boyd MB, McAllister KS, McDonald RA, et al. Afferent phase production of TNF-alpha is required for the development of protective T cell immunity to *Cryptococcus neoformans*. The Journal of Immunology. 1996;**157**:4529-4536

[83] Shourian M, Ralph B, Angers I, Sheppard DC, Qureshi ST. Contribution of IL-1RI signaling to protection against *Cryptococcus neoformans* 52D in a mouse model of infection. Frontiers in Immunology. 2018;**8**:1987

[84] Chen M, Xing Y, Lu A, Fang W, Sun B, Chen C, et al. Internalized *Cryptococcus neoformans* activates the canonical caspase-1 and the noncanonical caspase-8 inflammasomes. The Journal of Immunology. 2015;**195**(10):4962-4972

[85] Flesch I, Schwamberger G, Kaufmann S. Fungicidal activity of IFN-gamma-activated macrophages. Extracellular killing of *Cryptococcus neoformans*. The Journal of Immunology. 1989;**142**:3219-3224

[86] Chen G-H, McDonald RA, Wells JC, Huffnagle GB, Lukacs NW, Toews GB. The gamma interferon receptor is required for the protective pulmonary inflammatory response to *Cryptococcus neoformans*. Infection and Immunity. 2005;**73**:1788-1796

[87] Wager CML, Hole CR, Campuzano A, Castro-Lopez N, Cai H, Van Dyke MCC, et al. IFN-γ immune priming of macrophages in vivo induces prolonged STAT1 binding and protection against *Cryptococcus neoformans*. PLoS Pathogens. 2018;**14**:e1007358

[88] Wozniak KL, Hardison SE, Kolls JK, Wormley FL Jr. Role of IL-17A on resolution of pulmonary *C. neoformans* infection. PLoS One. 2011;**6**:e17204

[89] Wozniak KL, Hole CR, Yano J, Fidel PL Jr, Wormley FL Jr. Characterization of IL-22 and antimicrobial peptide production in mice protected against pulmonary *Cryptococcus neoformans* infection. Microbiology. 2014;**160**:1440-1452

[90] Aguirre K, Gibson G. Differing requirement for inducible nitric oxide synthase activity in clearance of primary and secondary *Cryptococcus neoformans* infection. Medical Mycology. 2000;**38**:343-353

[91] Osterholzer JJ, Chen G-H, Olszewski MA, Zhang Y-M, Curtis JL, Huffnagle GB, et al. Chemokine receptor 2-mediated accumulation of fungicidal exudate macrophages in mice that clear cryptococcal lung infection. The American Journal of Pathology. 2011;**178**:198-211

[92] Espinosa V, Jhingran A, Dutta O, Kasahara S, Donnelly R, Du P, et al. Inflammatory monocytes orchestrate innate antifungal immunity in the lung. PLoS Pathogens. 2014;**10**:e1003940

[93] Fa Z, Xie Q, Fang W, Zhang H, Xu J, Pan W, et al. RIPK3/Fas-associated death domain Axis regulates pulmonary Immunopathology to Cryptococcal infection independent of Necroptosis. Frontiers in Immunology. 2017;**8**:1055

[94] Zelante T, De Luca A, Bonifazi P, Montagnoli C, Bozza S, Moretti S, et al. IL-23 and the Th17 pathway promote inflammation and impair antifungal immune resistance. European Journal of Immunology. 2007;**37**:2695-2706

[95] Eastman AJ, Osterholzer JJ, Olszewski MA. Role of dendritic cell-pathogen interactions in the immune response to pulmonary cryptococcal infection. Future Microbiology. 2015;**10**:1837-1857

[96] Bonifazi P, Zelante T, D'angelo C, De Luca A, Moretti S, Bozza S, et al. Balancing inflammation and tolerance in vivo through dendritic cells by the commensal *Candida albicans*. Mucosal Immunology. 2009;**2**:362

[97] Osterholzer JJ, Milam JE, Chen G-H, Toews GB, Huffnagle GB, Olszewski MA. Role of dendritic cells and alveolar macrophages in regulating early host defense against pulmonary infection with *Cryptococcus neoformans*. Infection and Immunity. 2009;**77**:3749-3758

[98] Abraham E. Neutrophils and acute lung injury. Critical Care Medicine. 2003;**31**:S195-S199

[99] Esher SK, Zaragoza O, Alspaugh JA. Cryptococcal pathogenic mechanisms: A dangerous trip from the environment to the brain. Memórias do Instituto Oswaldo Cruz. 2018;**113**(7):e180057

[100] Arora S, Huffnagle GB. Immune regulation during allergic bronchopulmonary mycosis. Immunologic Research. 2005;**33**:53-68

[101] Greenberger PA, Bush RK, Demain JG, Luong A, Slavin RG, Knutsen AP. Allergic bronchopulmonary aspergillosis. The Journal of Allergy

and Clinical Immunology: In Practice. 2014;**2**:703-708

[102] Wiesner DL, Specht CA, Lee CK, Smith KD, Mukaremera L, Lee ST, et al. Chitin recognition via chitotriosidase promotes pathologic type-2 helper T cell responses to cryptococcal infection. PLoS Pathogens. 2015;**11**:e1004701

[103] Müller U, Stenzel W, Köhler G, Werner C, Polte T, Hansen G, et al. IL-13 induces disease-promoting type 2 cytokines, alternatively activated macrophages and allergic inflammation during pulmonary infection of mice with Cryptococcus neoformans. The Journal of Immunology. 2007;**179**:5367-5377

[104] Saenz SA, Taylor BC, Artis D. Welcome to the neighborhood: Epithelial cell-derived cytokines license innate and adaptive immune responses at mucosal sites. Immunological Reviews. 2008;**226**:172-190

[105] Liew FY, Pitman NI, McInnes IB. Disease-associated functions of IL-33: The new kid in the IL-1 family. Nature Reviews Immunology. 2010;**10**:103

[106] Flaczyk A, Duerr CU, Shourian M, Lafferty EI, Fritz JH, Qureshi ST. IL-33 signaling regulates innate and adaptive immunity to Cryptococcus neoformans. The Journal of Immunology. 2013;**191**(5):2503-2513

[107] Allen JE, Wynn TA. Evolution of Th2 immunity: A rapid repair response to tissue destructive pathogens. PLoS Pathogens. 2011;**7**:e1002003

[108] Arendse B, Schwegmann A, Radwanska M, Leeto M, Kirsch R, Hall P, et al. Alternative macrophage activation is essential for survival during schistosomiasis and downmodulates T helper 1 responses and immunopathology. Immunity. 2004;**21**:455

[109] Gallagher I, Nair MG, Zang X, Brombacher F, Mohrs M, Allison JP, et al. Alternative activation is an innate response to injury that requires CD4+ T cells to be sustained during chronic infection. The Journal of Immunology. 2007;**179**:3926-3936

[110] Sanjabi S, Zenewicz LA, Kamanaka M, Flavell RA. Anti-inflammatory and pro-inflammatory roles of TGF-β, IL-10, and IL-22 in immunity and autoimmunity. Current Opinion in Pharmacology. 2009;**9**:447-453

[111] Sakaguchi S. Naturally arising CD4+ regulatory T cells for immunologic self-tolerance and negative control of immune responses. Annual Review of Immunology. 2004;**22**:531-562

[112] Barnes MJ, Powrie F. Regulatory T cells reinforce intestinal homeostasis. Immunity. 2009;**31**:401-411

[113] Schulze B, Piehler D, Eschke M, von Buttlar H, Kohler G, Sparwasser T, et al. CD4(+) FoxP3(+) regulatory T cells suppress fatal T helper 2 cell immunity during pulmonary fungal infection. European Journal of Immunology. 2014;**44**:3596-3604

[114] Netea MG, Sutmuller R, Hermann C, Van der Graaf CA, Van der Meer JW, Van Krieken JH, et al. Toll-like receptor 2 suppresses immunity against Candida albicans through induction of IL-10 and regulatory T cells. The Journal of Immunology. 2004;**172**:3712-3718

[115] Montagnoli C, Fallarino F, Gaziano R, Bozza S, Bellocchio S, Zelante T, et al. Immunity and tolerance to Aspergillus involve functionally distinct regulatory T cells and tryptophan catabolism. The Journal of Immunology. 2006;**176**:1712-1723

[116] Wiesner DL, Smith KD, Kotov DI, Nielsen JN, Bohjanen PR, Nielsen K. Regulatory T cell induction and retention in the lungs drives

suppression of detrimental type 2 Th cells during pulmonary cryptococcal infection. Journal of Immunology. 2016;**196**:365-374

[117] De Luca A, Montagnoli C, Zelante T, Bonifazi P, Bozza S, Moretti S, et al. Functional yet balanced reactivity to Candida albicans requires TRIF, MyD88, and IDO-dependent inhibition of Rorc. The Journal of Immunology. 2007;**179**:5999-6008

[118] Whibley N, MacCallum DM, Vickers MA, Zafreen S, Waldmann H, Hori S, et al. Expansion of Foxp3+ T-cell populations by Candida albicans enhances both Th17-cell responses and fungal dissemination after intravenous challenge. European Journal of Immunology. 2014;**44**:1069-1083

[119] Belkaid Y, Tarbell K. Regulatory T cells in the control of host-microorganism interactions. Annual Review of Immunology. 2009;**27**:551-589

[120] Montagnoli C, Bacci A, Bozza S, Gaziano R, Mosci P, Sharpe AH, et al. B7/CD28-dependent CD4+ CD25+ regulatory T cells are essential components of the memory-protective immunity to Candida albicans. The Journal of Immunology. 2002;**169**:6298-6308

[121] McKinley L, Logar AJ, McAllister F, Zheng M, Steele C, Kolls JK. Regulatory T cells dampen pulmonary inflammation and lung injury in an animal model of pneumocystis pneumonia. The Journal of Immunology. 2006;**177**:6215-6226

[122] Hesse M, Piccirillo CA, Belkaid Y, Prufer J, Mentink-Kane M, Leusink M, et al. The pathogenesis of schistosomiasis is controlled by cooperating IL-10-producing innate effector and regulatory T cells. The Journal of Immunology. 2004;**172**:3157-3166

[123] Guilliams M, Oldenhove G, Noel W, Hérin M, Brys L, Loi P, et al. African trypanosomiasis: Naturally occurring regulatory T cells favor trypanotolerance by limiting pathology associated with sustained type 1 inflammation. The Journal of Immunology. 2007;**179**:2748-2757

[124] Schulze B, Piehler D, Eschke M, Heyen L, Protschka M, Köhler G, et al. Therapeutic expansion of CD4+ FoxP3+ regulatory T cells limits allergic airway inflammation during pulmonary fungal infection. FEMS Pathogens and Disease. 2016;**74**:ftw020

[125] Vignali DA, Collison LW, Workman CJ. How regulatory T cells work. Nature Reviews Immunology. 2008;**8**:523

[126] Couper KN, Blount DG, Riley EM. IL-10: The master regulator of immunity to infection. The Journal of Immunology. 2008;**180**:5771-5777

[127] Hernandez Y, Arora S, Erb-Downward JR, McDonald RA, Toews GB, Huffnagle GB. Distinct roles for IL-4 and IL-10 in regulating T2 immunity during allergic bronchopulmonary mycosis. The Journal of Immunology. 2005;**174**:1027-1036

[128] Murdock BJ, Teitz-Tennenbaum S, Chen GH, Dils AJ, Malachowski AN, Curtis JL, et al. Early or late IL-10 blockade enhances Th1 and Th17 effector responses and promotes fungal clearance in mice with cryptococcal lung infection. Journal of Immunology. 2014;**193**:4107-4116

[129] Vazquez-Torres A, Jones-Carson J, Wagner RD, Warner T, Balish E. Early resistance of interleukin-10 knockout mice to acute systemic candidiasis. Infection and Immunity. 1999;**67**:670-674

[130] Sahaza JH, Suárez-Alvarez R, Estrada-Bárcenas DA, Pérez-Torres A,

Taylor ML. Profile of cytokines in the lungs of BALB/c mice after intra-nasal infection with Histoplasma capsulatum mycelial propagules. Comparative Immunology, Microbiology and Infectious Diseases. 2015;**41**:1-9

[131] Mirkov I, Demenesku J, Aleksandrov AP, Ninkov M, Glamoclija J, Kataranovski D, et al. Strain differences in the immune mechanisms of resistance of immunocompetent rats to pulmonary aspergillosis. Immunobiology. 2015;**220**:1075-1084

[132] Kühn R, Löhler J, Rennick D, Rajewsky K, Müller W. Interleukin-10-deficient mice develop chronic enterocolitis. Cell. 1993;**75**:263-274

[133] Hoshi N, Schenten D, Nish SA, Walther Z, Gagliani N, Flavell RA, et al. MyD88 signalling in colonic mononuclear phagocytes drives colitis in IL-10-deficient mice. Nature Communications. 2012;**3**:1120

[134] Tan D, Yong Y, Tan H, Kamarulzaman A, Tan L, Lim A, et al. Immunological profiles of immune restoration disease presenting as mycobacterial lymphadenitis and cryptococcal meningitis. HIV Medicine. 2008;**9**:307-316

[135] Beardsley J, Wolbers M, Kibengo FM, Ggayi AB, Kamali A, Cuc NT, et al. Adjunctive dexamethasone in HIV-associated cryptococcal meningitis. The New England Journal of Medicine. 2016;**374**:542-554

[136] Jarvis JN, Meintjes G, Rebe K, Williams GN, Bicanic T, Williams A, et al. Adjunctive interferon-gamma immunotherapy for the treatment of HIV-associated cryptococcal meningitis: A randomized controlled trial. AIDS. 2012;**26**:1105-1113

Chapter 3

Invasive Candidiasis: Epidemiology and Risk Factors

Jorge Alberto Cortés and Ivohne Fernanda Corrales

Abstract

Invasive candidiasis is a severe infection caused by the yeast of the genus *Candida*. This highly lethal infection can affect any organs, but it is usually identified by the growth of the yeast in bloodstream samples. Although *C. albicans* was the most frequently found species, there has been a global trend to the non-albicans isolates. The appearance of *C. auris,* a newly identified species around the world, is a cause of concern because of resistance to antifungals. In this chapter, the epidemiology and risk factors for the acquisition of candidemia and other forms of invasive candidiasis are reviewed, while showing the current knowledge of worldwide epidemiology.

Keywords: *Candida*, *Candida albicans*, invasive, candidiasis, fungemia, candidemia, intensive care units, surgery, immunosuppression, microbiota

1. Introduction

Candidiasis is the common name for diseases produced by the yeast of the genus *Candida*. This is the most frequently found yeast in human microbiome and is capable of causing disease at different sites of the human anatomy and with diverse severity [1]. Invasive candidiasis refers to severe fungal infections in which the yeast might be found in deep organs or blood [2]. Due to the difficulty of identifying *Candida* yeasts in tissues, since it requires a biopsy of the tissue compromised, invasive candidiasis in the literature has been primarily found as bloodstream infections, alone or with accompanying tissue compromise.

2. Microbiology and environment

Candida species are yeasts (i.e., they mainly have a unicellular form). They are small, with a size of 4–6 μm, with a thin wall and an ovoid aspect, named blastospores [3]. They reproduce by budding. Using the microscope, these yeasts can be seen in the form of pseudohyphae, budding cells that do not separate, or truly hyphae (multicellular organisms). *Candida* organisms belong to the class Ascomycetes, order Saccharomycetales, and family Saccharomycetes [4]. There are around 200 species of *Candida;* however, a limited number has a pathogenic effect on humans [4]. **Table 1** shows the most frequently found species. Due to their previous prevalence and pathogenic significance, they were usually classified as *albicans*

Species	Characteristic
C. albicans	Usually the most frequently found
C. parapsilosis complex	*C. parapsilosis, C. orthopsilosis, C. metapsilosis*
C. tropicalis	Related to cancer
C. glabrata	Usually resistant to azoles, seen more frequently in developed scenarios and older patients
C. guilliermondii	Less pathogenicity
C. lusitaniae	Potentially resistant to amphotericin
C. krusei	Intrinsically resistant to azoles
C. dubliniensis	Difficult to differentiate from *C. albicans*
C. auris	Responsible for a global outbreak

Table 1.
Most frequently found Candida *species in human disease.*

versus *non-albicans Candida* species. However, due to changes in epidemiology, this overall classification might not be useful any more.

They grow in agar as colonies with a smooth, creamy, white appearance. The formal identification can be made by use of biochemical physiological reactions, which can differentiate an important number of isolates. The metabolic reactions include carbohydrate fermentation, nitrate use, and urease production.

Candida yeasts might be seen with direct stains like KOH with 10–20% concentrations, but also with others like Gram, Giemsa, Wright para amino-salicylic (PAS) acid, and Papanicolaou. In direct stains, *Candida* might be seen as big aggregates of blastoconidiae, with short and large pseudohyphae. Usual growth media include Sabouraud agar, brain infusion, heart, and yeast extract. While *C. albicans* and *C. dubliniensis* grow in usual Sabouraud agar with antibiotics, some species might be inhibited by cycloheximide [4]. Usual growth time is 2–3 days at 28–37°C. Chromogenic agars were developed more than 20 years ago and are capable of identifying the most commonly found species, and speciation is desirable due to pathogenic and susceptibility differences among them. There are several commercial methods using chromogenic agars. The sensitivity for detection of *Candida* yeast is over 95%, usually with a low number or no false positive results [5]. The finding of a positive culture does not imply an invasive infection, and a special consideration has to be made for isolates from sterile sites.

Candida species differ in their susceptibility to different antifungals available in different countries. Most frequently found isolates of *C. albicans* and *C. parapsilosis* are susceptible to all antifungals available. *C. tropicalis* might have some resistance to fluconazole, while maintaining susceptibility to equinocandins and amphotericin B. *C. glabrata* tends to have higher minimal inhibitory concentrations (MICs) to azoles, while remaining susceptible to equinocandins and amphotericin B. *C. lusitaniae* isolates can be found to be resistant to amphotericin B. The recently found that *C. auris* is frequently found multidrug resistant.

Susceptibility testing can be performed by different methods, including broth microdilution (recommended in the USA and Europe), but there are other different commercial methods available in hospitals. Two slightly different standards for susceptibility testing are currently available. One is suggested by the Clinical Laboratory Standards Institute (CLSI, in USA), while the other is proposed by the European Committee on Antimicrobial Susceptibility Testing (EUCAST), sponsored by the European Society of Clinical Microbiology and Infectious Diseases

(ESCMID). Basic differences between both methodologies include time and instrument to read the results. Different clinical breakpoints have been established for the most commonly found species, with the intention of differentiating the risk of clinical failure after treatment. The experience with fluconazole has allowed to develop better prediction models, in comparison with newer antifungals [6]. In summary, an isolate of *Candida* is exposed to different concentrations of the antifungal and the *in vitro* growth is observed. If there is no important growth, determined optically or by a spectrophotometer, a minimal inhibitory concentration (MIC) is established. As mentioned, data from clinical trials and observation cohorts with common species such as *C. albicans* and *C. glabrata* have allowed to identify clinically relevant breakpoints to differentiate isolates with low MICs (susceptible); intermediate MICs (also called susceptible dose dependent—SDD), in which an increase in the administered antifungal can control the infection; and high MICs, (resistant), for which a lower probability of success is expected. For some other uncommon species, only epidemiological breakpoints are available. These breakpoints are also MICs, but there is no clinical evidence of correlation with the clinical outcome after treatment. However, since MICs are higher than those in usual isolates, a worse outcome might be expected. These breakpoints are expected to identify isolates with natural or acquired mechanisms of antifungal resistance. The epidemiological breakpoints are based on the statistical distribution of MICs of the wild-type isolates (i.e., isolates without any previous resistant pressure). Commercial methods are modifications of the standard methods that use dyes to identify the growth (e.g., Alamar Blue) of the microorganisms. Examples include Sensititre™ and YeastOne™. Other methods are based on agar, in which a gradient of the antifungal is diffused in the solid growth media, which allows to directly read the MIC (e.g., Etest ™) [7].

Candida species are part of the human microbiota and they live in human mucosae and skin. *Candida* species can be found in the ground, animals, fruits and vegetables, and in the hospital environment. It is not considered a laboratory contaminant. It is considered an endogenous pathogen since around 60–75% of the people might have it in the mucosal epithelium, especially in the gastrointestinal and genital tracts [8]. In the hospital area, they have been found over inanimate surfaces, including percutaneous catheters and tubes. They might even be found in the hands of healthcare workers. Among patients in healthcare centers, the colonization of the mucosae has been related to antibiotic use and hospitalization time [9]. In patients in the intensive care unit (ICU), colonization might be found in different anatomical sites with ample variations [10, 11]. Pharyngeal colonization rate has been found to be between 34 and 65%, gastric colonization between 42 and 67%, rectal colonization between 21 and 40%, and colonization in other sites between 11 and 40% [10, 11]. These data show the possibility of colonization that has this microorganism in patients under stress conditions (in this case, severe disease). In the normal host, the colonization rate might reach over 50% in the mouth, 40% in the vaginal tissue in women, and 73% in any mucosa of the gastrointestinal or genital tracts [8].

3. Pathogenesis

Candida species have some characteristics that permit them to adapt to different environments and act as an opportunistic pathogen. These factors include adaptation to pH changes, permitting to survive in blood or some alkaline environments, as well as in the acidic environment of the vaginal tissue; these species have adhesins, mannoproteins with capacity to adhere to different cells and cell products.

These adherence proteins allow the isolates to survive in tissues, but also over inanimate surfaces that have been exposed to plasma or inflammatory host proteins like urinary or endotracheal catheters. *Candida* species have also important enzymes as virulence factors, since some of them have keratinolytic, peptidase, hemolysin, and other effects. One of the most frequently mentioned virulence factors include the possibility of a morphologic transition, which has been extensively studied. It refers to the possibility of morphologic changes of blastoconidia to pseudohyphae to real hyphae. These changes are stimulated by environmental conditions. The filamentous forms are related to active infection in the host, except for *C. glabrata*. Other factors related to pathogenicity or virulence also include a phenotyping change, the possibility of adopting different phenotypes in the cultures (color or aspect of the colonies), and biofilm formation. A biofilm is a large community of symbiotic microorganisms adhered to a surface. This conformation allows the microorganisms to have a highly defensive capacity, persistence, and a highly antimicrobial resistance.

As mentioned before, *Candida* might be part of the human flora. The majority of infections are due to the interplay between the risk factors, that pose a risk to the individual, the interaction with other microorganisms present in the skin or mucosa and the total quantity of microorganisms present. This was demonstrated some years ago in an experiment [12]. An individual ingested directly from a *C. albicans* culture. After some hours, this immunocompetent individual began to have fever. After 12 hours, *Candida* isolates were found in the bloodstream and, after 16 hours, they were found in the urine. After 24 hours, *Candida* isolates were cleared from the body and the individual returned to the normal state. This experiment proved the importance of colonization. With posterior evidence, it has been demonstrated that the first step to have an infection is colonization by *Candida* especially in the gastrointestinal tract, but otherwise in contact with indwelling catheters, the skin, or wounds that may permit the entry of the yeast into the bloodstream. In another critical observation, patients in the ICU were followed with cultures. The colonization index (it is the proportion of positive cultures for the same *Candida* species taken from different anatomical places) increased over time and was correlated to the probability of developing an invasive candidiasis [9]. These studies suggest that in individuals with *Candida* colonization, those factors that promote the grow of the yeast, by eliminating the bacteria that can compete for the environment, that alter or facilitate the penetration of the yeast to the bloodstream (lesions in the gastrointestinal mucosa, indwelling catheters) will promote the entry of *Candida* yeast to the blood, while the net state of compromise of the immune system will affect the probability of fungal clearance and the possibility of seeding on specific organs.

4. Epidemiology

4.1 Risk factors

4.1.1 Candida infection in the intensive care unit

Patients in the ICU have the highest rate of *Candida* infections in the hospital. In comparison with patients in other wards, patients in the ICU have more frequent abdominal surgery, stay longer in the hospital, and are more severely ill [13]. They also have a worse prognosis in the long term, with increased mortality after one year of the event.

4.1.1.1 Vascular devices

Patients in the ICU have higher rates of *Candida* infection in comparison with patients in other wards. Critically ill patients often require multiple vascular and other indwelling devices for their management and candidemia has been related to catheter colonization in 20–80% of the cases [14, 15]. One study in Japan identified the presence of a solid tumor, the use of total parenteral nutrition, and the administration of anti-anaerobic agents as the main risk factors for the development of *Candida* infections [16]. As mentioned, *Candida* colonization of the catheter might provide a route for entering into the bloodstream without a heavy gastrointestinal colonization. Studies have shown that *Candida* catheter-related bloodstream infections have a shorter time to grow in comparison with those from other sources [14]. With a breakpoint of 30 hours, the time to grow in patients with *Candida* bloodstream infection might identify 100% of those catheter-related infection. Probably, patients with catheter-related infection have a higher inoculum, which would explain the faster time to grow and the fact that observational studies have shown a lower mortality when catheter is removed [17, 18]. On the other hand, patients with non-catheter-related candidemia were more seriously ill, had a higher mortality, and the removal of the catheter did not affect the outcome [17].

4.1.1.2 Parenteral nutrition

Another commonly identified risk factor is the use of parenteral nutrition or the length of its use [15, 19]. This group of patients shares several risk factors, but parenteral nutrition has been identified in multivariate analysis [20]. Usually, they have an abdominal procedure (see below) and they require parenteral nutrition for several days. Lack of appropriate measures to handle the nutrition, colonization of the catheter or the ports used to infuse it, and probably the availability of optimal growing conditions are conditions related to its use. But clearly, the use of parenteral nutrition leads to the development of mucosal atrophy and a loss of mucosal epithelial barrier function [21], which might affect the relationship between microorganisms in the gut and the possibility of gaining access to blood vessels. Total parenteral nutrition has also a profound effect in the gastrointestinal microbiome [22].

4.1.1.3 Surgical procedures

Several studies have shown the relationship between candidemia and a previous surgical procedure [19, 23], specially an abdominal surgery. There are several explanations to this observation, but gut manipulation, and the effect of resected sections over the gut microbiology, microbiota abundance, and epithelial function might contribute to the possibility of candidemia. Studies have shown that patients with high anastomotic leak, as well as those with recurrent gastrointestinal perforation, or acute necrotizing pancreatitis, have a higher risk of candidemia [15].

4.1.1.4 Antibiotic use

Almost all studies of candidemia have shown an extremely high use of antibiotics previous to the identification of bloodstream or tissue infection. The proportion of patients with antibiotic use is over 80% [24]. The number and spectrum of the antibiotics used might affect the risk of candidemia. Antimicrobials also have an effect over gut microbiota, and some studies have shown some impact from antibiotics with anti-anaerobic effect, and those with higher gastrointestinal concentration [25]. They contribute to the observed increased colonization over time observed in patients in the ICU. With more antibiotic effect, there is a net decrease in the number of species in the gastrointestinal tract, an increase in the number of patients colonized, and the proportion of them being heavily colonized [26].

4.1.1.5 Other risk factors

Studies have identified several risk factors that alone, or in combination, might increase the probability of having candidemia. The presence of renal failure, the use of antihistaminic blockers, the severity of illness, and the length of stay in the ICU contribute to colonization and development of candidemia [24, 27]. All these factors contribute to the acquisition of *Candida*, its colonization, or failure in the gastrointestinal epithelial function, favoring the entry of the yeast to the bloodstream.

4.1.1.6 Scores based on risk factors

The identification of risk factors lead to the use of some scores based in the presence of such factors to identify patients with higher risk of *Candida* infection. The first and most simple of those scores was introduced in mid-1990s. Pittet et al. in a surgical ICU followed prospectively patients admitted in the ward with cultures of several anatomical sites [9]. They defined the colonization index as previously stated, establishing that with an index of 0.5 or more (50% of the sites with the same species), there was an increase in the risk of candidemia. With a lower colonization index, the risk in the original study was 0%. They defined a second index based on the density of colonization, in which patients overpassing some thresholds in the number of colonies isolated per site, being able to improve the identification of the patients at risk.

A second score to identify risk factors in patients was developed in Spain by León and his collaborators [20]. They identified colonization (with a different definition from that used by Pittet et al.), surgery at ICU admission, and use of total parenteral nutrition as risk factors independently associated with candidemia. They also identified sepsis as independently related, but this is clearly more a clinical syndrome than a risk factor. A third score was developed by a multicenter collaboration group, in which they again identified the same risk factors [28]: antibiotic use, having an intravascular catheter, in conjunction with at least two additional risk factors such as any surgery, immunosuppressive use, pancreatitis, total parenteral nutrition, dialysis, or steroid use.

Common to these scores has been the presence of the aforementioned risk factors. The problem, however, is that such scores identify a huge number of patients at risk with a final intermediate risk of developing candidemia, in a range from 7 to 30% [29, 30]. The great advantage of the diagnostic scores relies in their high negative predictive value. Patients with a negative score have a low probability of candidemia, below a 1% probability.

4.1.2 Hematological malignancy, solid organ transplantation, and other immunosuppressive states

These disorders share a common factor: immunosuppression. However, different types of immunocompromise entail different risks for the patients. The incidence of candidemia among patients with cancer is higher in comparison with other patients in the hospital. In a multicenter study in Greece, patients with hematological disease had an incidence of candidemia of 1.4 cases per 1000 admissions, while other patients hospitalized had an incidence of 0.83 cases per 1000 admissions [31]. A multicenter European study found an incidence of 1.2% cases of candidemia among patients with bone marrow transplantation (BMT) and leukemia [32]. An Italian multicenter study from a surveillance network showed a diminishing trend for candidemia among patients with cancer, especially among those with acute myeloid leukemia [33]. Whether this trend can be inferred to other European countries or not is not known, and the most likely explanation for this decrease in the number of cases could be related to the use of prophylaxis among those patients with acute leukemia with posaconazole. In general, non-albicans *Candida* species are more frequently found among these groups of patients [31].

4.1.2.1 Neutropenia

Neutropenia, a count of leukocytes in peripheral blood below 500 cells per μl, is the common risk factor among patients with hematological disorders (i.e., leukemia, lymphoma, multiple myeloma among others) as well as those with bone marrow transplantation (BMT). Neutropenia might be a consequence of the activity of the hematological disease, an effect of chemotherapeutic strategies or side effect of multiple medications including antimicrobials. It also is a marker of the intensity of chemotherapy. Patients with chemotherapy-induced neutropenia accumulate various risk factors: they usually receive wide spectrum antibiotics for several days, they have serious gastrointestinal epithelial tissue dysfunction, usually with diarrhea and signs of mucosal damage, and the use of vascular catheters for the infusion of chemotherapeutic drugs and antibiotics [34]. Several studies have shown that isolates of *C. tropicalis* are more frequently found among patients with cancer [35]. A study that looked for risk factors identified underlying leukemia as one of the major risk factors, together with chronic lung disease [36].

In patients with prolonged neutropenia, a condition called hepatosplenic candidiasis might be seen. In it, seeding of yeasts occurs during the neutropenic phase which might be not clinically evident until neutropenia recovery. In these patients, fever persists and lesions can be seen in the liver, usually known as bull-eye lesions [37] (**Figure 1**).

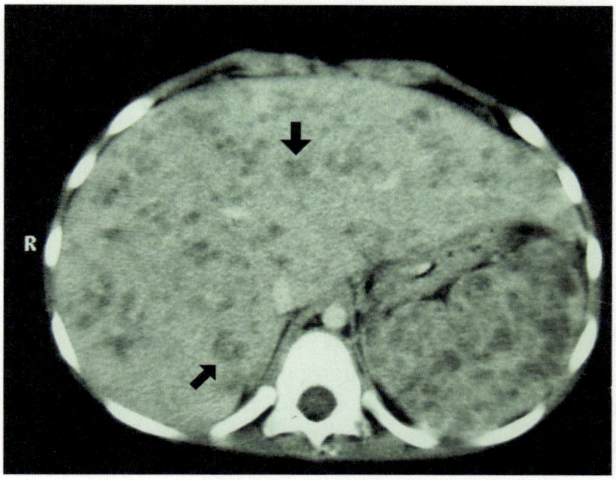

Figure 1.
Tomographic image of liver and spleen showing abscesses (bull's eye, arrows) and hypodense lesions in a patient with chronic disseminated candidiasis. Reproduced with permission from Cortés et al. [37].

4.1.2.2 Concurrent conditions in patients with cancer

In patients with cancer and candidemia, several factors were identified in comparison with those with cancer and bacterial infections [38]. Total parenteral nutrition over 5 days, urinary catheter for more than 2 days, distant metastasis of cancer, and gastrointestinal cancer were independent risk factors. Patients with solid tumors might accumulate factors as patients in critical care, since they have abdominal surgery (gastrointestinal neoplasm), require vascular catheters for extended periods of time (for chemotherapy or antibiotics), total parenteral nutrition and received antibiotics frequently [39]. A study to identify factors predicting catheter-related infections with *Candida* identified solid tumors and the use of anti-anaerobic antibiotics as risk factors [16].

Among patients with leukemia and BMT, the risk factors for occurrence of candidemia included bone marrow or cord blood stem cell source, T-cell depletion, use of total body irradiation, and acute graft versus host disease [32]. These data were derived from a huge multicenter registry of patients with cancer and transplantation, which allowed to identify more precisely the risk factors.

4.1.3 Neonates

Newborns have no gastrointestinal flora at birth and have to be colonized by enterobacteria and other microorganisms, which is made via maternal breast feeding. Any alteration in the normal process can lead to colonization by pathogenic microorganisms, including yeasts [40]. Neonates in the intensive care unit usually have limited breastfeeding, indwelling vascular catheters, total parenteral nutrition, and antibiotics [41]. Such combination of risk factors put. this group of patients at a higer risk of infection, reaching over 10% of patients in units with extreme prematures and low weight at birth (the group that requires more invasive interventions) [42]. Some studies have illustrated this relationship with proportion of candidemia between 3 and 10% among those with a weight of less than 1000 g while showing an incidence of less than 1% for those weighting over 2500 g [43]. In this scenario, disseminated candidemia can be found and near 10% of those with invasive disease can compromise the central nervous system. Another important risk factor includes the time that the patient has been in the unit [44]; clearly, patients with low weight, lower gestational age, and more comorbidity tend to spend more time in the neonatal ICU and to accumulate other risk factors (surgery, indwelling catheter, antibiotics, etc.) [45]. There are some high-risk units, in which the incidence of candidemia traditionally has been high, usually over 10% of the admitted cases. In this scenario, prophylaxis has been suggested for the prevention of infection [46].

4.1.4 Outbreaks

Candida yeast can survive in inanimate surfaces and in the hands of healthcare personnel, which confers the risk of outbreak and cross dissemination among high-risk units such as neonatal, intensive care, and surgical intensive care units [44, 47]. An interesting study in Iceland over a long period of time allowed to confirm the presence of clonal isolates of different *Candida* species among patients in the ICU and other wards [48]. The proportion of patients involved at one time with an outbreak of all patients with *Candida* isolates might be as high as 38%. Other study in Spain showed that clusters (of patients with candidemia) were possible with *C. albicans* and *C. parapsilosis*, and reached in a period as high as 40% of the isolates [49]. Besides, the use of chlorhexidine has been shown to diminish the number of candidemia events in patients in the ICU, showing the importance of colonization and cross infection among high-risk patients and establishing this recommendation in the guidelines for the prevention of candidemia [50].

As shown, colonization is the preliminary step to infection. Besides, a number of interventions are common to immunosuppressed and critically ill patients including indwelling catheters (urinary and vascular), severity of illness, total parenteral nutrition, etc. These conditions predispose the patients to cross contamination. An outbreak among newborns was demonstrated to be due to poor practices of catheter ports disinfection [51].

A study in China in a cancer institute showed that 21 out of 36 episodes of candidemia were caused by two endemic genotypes [52]. In this study, gastrointestinal cancer and insertion of a nasogastric tube were related to infection. As mentioned before, cancer patients with solid and hematological tumors share several of the risk factors of colonization and infection.

4.2 Global epidemiology

Since 2013, the Leading International Fungal Education (LIFE) portal has facilitated an important effort to know the epidemiology and burden of fungal infections around the world and allowed a better understanding of their epidemiology in different countries [53]. The real incidence of candidemia is difficult to calculate due to differences in the approach. While studies based on hospitals might overestimate the importance of some groups of high-risk patients, they are difficult to compare. Data from population studies might reflect better the real situation, but this kind of information is scarce. Studies have shown ample differences in the incidence in some regions and at specific times [54].

4.2.1 Changing trend for non-albicans Candida

Traditionally, *C. albicans* had been the most frequently isolated species. However, a trend toward non-albicans species has been observed around the world in the last 15 years. In United States, *C. glabrata* has been identified as second in frequency, while *C. parapsilosis* or *C. tropicalis* dispute this place in other regions. **Table 2** shows the proportion of isolates in some studies around the world in the last 10 years [55–59].

Two studies deserve a detailed description. The first one is a multicenter study from the Southeast Asia region, including 25 hospitals from 6 countries: China, Hong Kong, India, Singapore, Taiwan, and Thailand [60]. They found differences between the countries that include the frequency of *C. tropicalis* isolation, being

Area and publication year	*C. albicans* (%)	*C. glabrata* (%)	*C. tropicalis*	*C. parapsilosis*	References
USA 2012	38	29	17	10	[49]
Latin America 2013	37.6	6.3	17.6	26.5	[48]
Spain 2014	45.4	13.4	7.7	24.9	[50]
Asia-Pacific region 2016	20–55	5–22	2–20	8–27	[51]
France 2014	56	18.6	9.3	11.5	[52]

Table 2.
Proportion of Candida *species in selected studies of candidemia around the world.*

more commonly found in hematology-oncology wards and in tropical areas. This study confirmed the observed trend for a lower frequency of *C. albicans* isolates. The other study is the Latin-American surveillance study [55]. It involved patients from 20 centers in 7 seven countries: Argentina, Brazil, Colombia, Chile, Honduras, Mexico, and Venezuela. Important differences were seen among institutions, reflecting difference in healthcare systems, access, population types, and risk factors. However, in these two studies, the incidence of candidemia is higher than in developed countries in Europe and North America. In Latin America, *C. parapsilosis* frequency is over 30% of the isolates while this place is occupied by *C. tropicalis* in the Asian countries.

4.2.2 Epidemiology in Europe and North America

There are data from some population surveillance surveys in Europe and United States. In general, the incidence might be lower than in some other areas of the world. **Table 3** shows the incidence from data from North America and European countries [61–77]. In Europe, the highest incidence has been observed in Hungary, while in North America the highest incidence has been seen in some cities in United States.

4.2.3 Epidemiology in Central and South America and the Caribbean

This region has profound differences in healthcare systems, access to care, and medical technology development. With a transition toward a higher income, a growing number of institutions with capacity to attend cancer patients, and more

Country/region	Publication Year	Incidence (per 100.000 inhabitants)	References
Belgium	2015	5	[54]
Denmark	2008	10.4	[55]
Finland	2010	2.8	[56]
Germany	2015	4.6	[57]
Hungary	2015	11	[58]
Ireland	2015	7.3	[59]
Norway	2018	3.8	[60]
Portugal	2017	2.57	[61]
Romania	2018	6.8	[62]
Russia	2015	8.29	[63]
Serbia	2018	10	[64]
Spain	2015	8.1	[65]
Sweden	2013	4.2	[66]
Ukraine	2015	5.8	[67]
Canada	2017	2.91	[68]
México	2015	8.6	[69]
USA	2015	9.5–14.4	[70]

Table 3.
Estimated incidence of invasive candidiasis or candidemia in countries of the European or North American regions.

Country/region	Publication year	Incidence (per 100,000 inhabitants)	References
Argentina	2018	6.25	[71]
Brazil	2016	14.9	[72]
Chile	2017	5.8	[73]
Colombia	2018	14.7	[74]
Ecuador	2017	7.2	[75]
Guatemala	2017	6.4	[76]
Jamaica	2015	5.8	[77]
Perú	2017	5.8	[78]
Trinidad and Tobago	2015	5.8	[79]
Uruguay	2018	36.5	[80]

Table 4.
Estimated incidence of invasive candidiasis or candidemia in countries of Central and South America and the Caribbean.

complex medical needs, the number of candidemia cases seems to be higher than in developed countries.

Ample information exists about the problem in Brazil, where a number of studies have been carried out in high-complexity hospitals in the main cities of the country [78, 79]. These studies show a higher frequency of invasive candidiasis in comparison with developed countries, an increased isolation of *C. glabrata* for the last period and an important exposition to fluconazole (which might have increased the selection for non-albicans species) [79]. Country-wise estimates for incidence are shown in **Table 4** [80–89].

4.2.4 Epidemiology in Africa and Asia

A multicenter in Asia gathered information from various countries, including nine hospitals from China [60]. The incidence rate among patients hospitalized was 0.38 per 1000 admissions, which is lower than that observed in the Latin-American region with 1.08 cases per 1000 admissions [55]. The estimated incidence of candidemia in countries in Asia is shown in **Table 5** [90–100]. In Asia, the highest incidence has been observed in Pakistan, followed by Qatar and Israel. In China, geographic variations in the causative species and susceptibilities were noted, with increasing isolates resistant to fluconazole [101]. The numbers for the African countries are lacking and for some countries like Algeria, Burkina Faso, Cameroon, Egypt, Malawi, Mozambique, and Tanzania, the estimated incidence is 5.8 cases per 100,000 inhabitants, a standard calculation based on previously reported incidence in other countries [102–108].

4.2.5 Azole resistance epidemiology

Azole-resistant *Candida* isolates have had an increased frequency over the years. Susceptibility changes with the species, and fluconazole use has been related to an increase in the frequency of *C. glabrata* and *C. krusei,* and a low increase in the number of resistant *C. albicans* or *C. tropicalis*. A large multicenter study in French ICUs identified the age and the exposure to antifungals as independent risk factors for resistance [109]. Patients with isolates resistant to fluconazole tended to be older than 15 years and to have been exposed to this drug, while those with

Country/region	Publication year	Incidence (per 100,000 inhabitants)	References
Bangladesh	2017	5	[83]
Israel	2015	11	[84]
Jordan	2018	5.75	[85]
Kazakhstan	2018	4.3	[86]
Korea	2017	4.57	[87]
Malaysia	2018	5.8	[88]
Pakistan	2017	21	[89]
Philippines	2017	2.25	[90]
Qatar	2015	15.4	[91]
Thailand	2015	13.3	[92]
Uzbekistan	2017	5.93	[93]

Table 5.
Estimated incidence of invasive candidiasis or candidemia in countries of Africa and Asia.

equinocandin-resistant isolates were younger and found to have been exposed to equinocandin. In general, risk factors for resistance remain the same as in resistant bacteria: immunosuppression, previous use of antifungals [110, 111]. Other identified risk factors include chronic renal failure and anti-tuberculous treatment. This last one might be due to a medication interaction.

Among patients with cancer, not only are non-albicans *Candida* species more frequently found, but also resistance to azoles has increased. In a study in Greece, resistance to fluconazole among patients with cancer reached 27% [31]. Since azoles have been widely used in the prophylaxis against fungal infections among cancer patients [112, 113], this seems to be a natural consequence of their use. Among patients with cancer, isolates of *C. tropicalis*, *C. glabrata*, and *C. krusei* have increased resistant proportions [35].

4.2.6 Candida auris *global outbreak*

Up to 2009, there was no report on *C. auris*. In that year, a clinical case from Japan was published, and 2 years later three cases of candidemia were identified [114, 115]. During the following years, isolates of *C. auris* were responsible of outbreaks around the world, affecting hospitals in India, Pakistan, South Africa, England, and Venezuela [116–119]. It was detected in the USA in 2013 with growing frequency [120]. A worldwide alarm was raised in 2016 because of two problems related to this species. The first one was the difficulty in proper identification [121]. *C. auris* is most commonly identified as *C. haemulonii* and *Rhodotorula glutinis* by the commercial systems and sometimes as *C. famata*, *C. guilliermondii*, and *C. parapsilosis* [121]. The other problem is the higher frequency of resistance to multiple antifungals, including azoles and amphotericin [122]. Currently, *C. auris* has been isolated in several areas in the USA, continental Europe, and the Caribbean coast of South America, including the islands [123–125], and continue to extend to other areas, where reports are being published. A search for virulence factors in the isolates of *C. auris* has shown some different properties, specially the capacity for biofilm formation [126]. Molecular observations have diverse geographic dissemination caused by unique clades in each geographic region [127].

5. Outcomes

Patients with candidemia and cancer are considered to have higher mortality, but this issue has not been clearly assessed. Older studies showed an attributable mortality around 40%. Although mortality among patients with candidemia or invasive candidiasis is reported usually around 40–50%, they occur in patients with important comorbidity. A recent multicenter analysis showed a crude mortality for patients with candidemia of 53%, while those without candidemia had a mortality of 26% [128]. After adjusting in a propensity score analysis, the crude mortality was 51% for the candidemic patients and 37% for the others and the difference was not statistically significant. The study shows that an increase in mortality might exist for those patients with candidemia, but it is clear that patients with candidemia also have severe comorbidity and some of them can die with candidemia instead of because of it.

Risk factors for mortality among patients with candidemia include ascites, presence of septic shock, ICU admission, concomitant bacterial infection and catheter-related infections [129]. Studies with diverse population have shown that elderly patients have higher mortality [130]. In these patients, a combination of comorbidity, poor clinical situation, and more pathogenic species might contribute to their mortality [131]. A pooled analysis from patients included in randomized clinical trials comparing micafungin and amphotericin B showed differences among geographic regions, severity of disease (measured with Apache score for patients critically ill), and catheter removal [132]. In those with abdominal candidiasis, the lack of control of the source of infection has been related to increased risk of death [133]. Among patients with cancer, risk factor for mortality includes infection by a *C. tropicalis* isolate, a high Charlson index score, neutropenia, and septic shock [35, 134]. One multicenter study identified tachypnea as a risk factor for mortality [135], while others identified respiratory failure and use of non-antifungal medications [39]. Besides, antifungal prophylaxis and remission of the underlying cancer had a protective effect over mortality [135].

The impact of the antifungal treatment in the mortality of patients with candidemia is not entirely clear. There are several constrains to identify the benefits of the antifungal treatment: An important proportion of patients did not receive antifungal treatment despite the identification of a bloodstream infection; of those that receive the treatment, some of them can receive it as empirical treatment, based on the risk factors, clinical condition, while others have an antifungal started upon detection of candidemia. Besides, some of them are infected with a resistant isolate and some do poorly, and an additional antifungal must be started. Although meta-analysis with patient-level data has showed the benefit of equinocandin use (in contrast to azole treatment) [136], neither the cohort data [137], nor the randomized trials have confirmed this finding [138]. There is an additional complication in understanding this relationship; the laboratory breakpoints for identification of susceptible versus resistant isolates have changed over the time, especially for azoles [130]. Among those patients with septic shock, the delay in the administration of the antifungal treatment has been associated with increased mortality.

6. Conclusion

Candidemia is the most frequently found form of invasive candidiasis. The *Candida* species might be found as part of the flora and patients with previous colonization are at risk of developing an infection. They share some common factors like antibiotic exposure, use of indwelling catheters, parenteral nutrition, and surgery. These factors affect the normal physiology of the gastrointestinal tract or provide access to the bloodstream to yeast in patients with some comorbidities, in critical care or with immunosuppressive states.

Conflict of interest

There is no conflict of interest to declare.

Author details

Jorge Alberto Cortés[1*] and Ivohne Fernanda Corrales[2]

1 Department of Internal Medicine, School of Medicine, Universidad Nacional de Colombia, Bogotá, Colombia

2 Neonatal Intensive Care Unit, Fundación CardioInfantil, Bogotá, Colombia

*Address all correspondence to: jacortesl@unal.edu.co

References

[1] Kullberg BJ, Arendrup MC. Invasive candidiasis. The New England Journal of Medicine. 2015;**373**:1445-1456

[2] Quindos G. Epidemiology of candidaemia and invasive candidiasis. A changing face. Revista Iberoamericana de Micología. 2014;**31**:42-48

[3] Dadar M, Tiwari R, Karthik K, Chakraborty S, Shahali Y, Dhama K. *Candida albicans*—Biology, molecular characterization, pathogenicity, and advances in diagnosis and control—An update. Microbial Pathogenesis. 2018; **117**:128-138

[4] Howell SA, Hazen KC, Brandt ME. *Candida, Cryptococcus*, and other yeast of medical importance. En: Jorgensen JH, Pfaller MA, editors. Manual of Clinical Microbiology. Washington, D.C.: American Society of Microbiology. 2015:1984-2014

[5] Perry JD. A decade of development of chromogenic culture media for clinical microbiology in an era of molecular diagnostics. Clinical Microbiology Reviews. 2017;**30**:449-479

[6] Patel TS, Carver PL, Eschenauer GA. Are in vitro susceptibilities to azole antifungals predictive of clinical outcome in the treatment of candidemia? Journal of Clinical Microbiology. 2018

[7] Sanguinetti M, Posteraro B. Susceptibility testing of Fungi to antifungal drugs. Journal of Fungi (Basel). 2018;**4**:E110

[8] Odds FC. Candida infections: An overview. Critical Reviews in Microbiology. 1987;**15**:1-5

[9] Pittet D, Monod M, Suter PM, Frenk E, Auckenthaler R. Candida colonization and subsequent infections in critically ill surgical patients. Annals of Surgery. 1994;**220**:751-758

[10] Magill SS, Swoboda SM, Johnson EA, Merz WG, Pelz RK, Lipsett PA, et al. The association between anatomic site of Candida colonization, invasive candidiasis, and mortality in critically ill surgical patients. Diagnostic Microbiology and Infectious Disease. 2006;**55**:293-301

[11] Leon C, Alvarez-Lerma F, Ruiz-Santana S, Leon MA, Nolla J, Jorda R, et al. Fungal colonization and/or infection in non-neutropenic critically ill patients: Results of the EPCAN observational study. European Journal of Clinical Microbiology & Infectious Diseases. 2009;**28**:233-242

[12] Krause W, Matheis H, Wulf K. Fungaemia and funguria after oral administration of *Candida albicans*. Lancet. 1969;**1**:598-599

[13] Ylipalosaari P, Ala-Kokko TI, Karhu J, Koskela M, Laurila J, Ohtonen P, et al. Comparison of the epidemiology, risk factors, outcome and degree of organ failures of patients with candidemia acquired before or during ICU treatment. Critical Care. 2012;**16**:R62

[14] Ben-Ami R, Weinberger M, Orni-Wasserlauff R, Schwartz D, Itzhaki A, Lazarovitch T, et al. Time to blood culture positivity as a marker for catheter-related candidemia. Journal of Clinical Microbiology. 2008;**46**: 2222-2226

[15] Blumberg HM, Jarvis WR, Soucie JM, Edwards JE, Patterson JE, Pfaller MA, et al. Risk factors for candidal bloodstream infections in surgical intensive care unit patients: The NEMIS prospective multicenter study. The

National Epidemiology of Mycosis Survey. Clinical Infectious Diseases. 2001;**33**:177-186

[16] Nagao M, Hotta G, Yamamoto M, Matsumura Y, Ito Y, Takakura S, et al. Predictors of Candida spp. as causative agents of catheter-related bloodstream infections. Diagnostic Microbiology and Infectious Disease. 2014;**80**:200-203

[17] Arias S, Denis O, Montesinos I, Cherifi S, Miendje Deyi VY, Zech F. Epidemiology and mortality of candidemia both related and unrelated to the central venous catheter: A retrospective cohort study. European Journal of Clinical Microbiology & Infectious Diseases. 2017;**36**:501-507

[18] Garnacho-Montero J, Diaz-Martin A, Garcia-Cabrera E, Ruiz Perez de Pipaon M, Hernandez-Caballero C, Lepe-Jimenez JA. Impact on hospital mortality of catheter removal and adequate antifungal therapy in Candida spp. bloodstream infections. The Journal of Antimicrobial Chemotherapy. 2013; **68**:206-213

[19] Chow JK, Golan Y, Ruthazer R, Karchmer AW, Carmeli Y, Lichtenberg DA, et al. Risk factors for albicans and non-albicans candidemia in the intensive care unit. Critical Care Medicine. 2008;**36**:1993-1998

[20] Leon C, Ruiz-Santana S, Saavedra P, Almirante B, Nolla-Salas J, Alvarez-Lerma F, et al. A bedside scoring system ("Candida score") for early antifungal treatment in nonneutropenic critically ill patients with Candida colonization. Critical Care Medicine. 2006;**34**:730-737

[21] Yang H, Feng Y, Sun X, Teitelbaum DH. Enteral versus parenteral nutrition: Effect on intestinal barrier function. Annals of the New York Academy of Sciences. 2009;**1165**:338-346

[22] Pierre JF. Gastrointestinal immune and microbiome changes during parenteral nutrition. American Journal of Physiology. Gastrointestinal and Liver Physiology. 2017;**312**:G246-GG56

[23] Ortiz Ruiz G, Osorio J, Valderrama S, Alvarez D, Elias Diaz R, Calderon J, et al. Risk factors for candidemia in non-neutropenic critical patients in Colombia. Medicina Intensiva. 2016;**40**: 139-144

[24] Wey SB, Mori M, Pfaller MA, Woolson RF, Wenzel RP. Risk factors for hospital-acquired candidemia. A matched case-control study. Archives of Internal Medicine. 1989;**149**:2349-2353

[25] Samonis G, Gikas A, Anaissie EJ, Vrenzos G, Maraki S, Tselentis Y, et al. Prospective evaluation of effects of broad-spectrum antibiotics on gastrointestinal yeast colonization of humans. Antimicrobial Agents and Chemotherapy. 1993;**37**:51-53

[26] Guyton K, Alverdy JC. The gut microbiota and gastrointestinal surgery. Nature Reviews. Gastroenterology & Hepatology. 2017;**14**:43-54

[27] Bross J, Talbot GH, Maislin G, Hurwitz S, Strom BL. Risk factors for nosocomial candidemia: A case-control study in adults without leukemia. The American Journal of Medicine. 1989;**87**: 614-620

[28] Ostrosky-Zeichner L, Sable C, Sobel J, Alexander BD, Donowitz G, Kan V, et al. Multicenter retrospective development and validation of a clinical prediction rule for nosocomial invasive candidiasis in the intensive care setting. European Journal of Clinical Microbiology & Infectious Diseases. 2007;**26**:271-276

[29] Ostrosky-Zeichner L, Shoham S, Vazquez J, Reboli A, Betts R, Barron MA, et al. MSG-01: A randomized, double-blind, placebo-controlled trial of caspofungin prophylaxis followed by preemptive therapy for invasive

candidiasis in high-risk adults in the critical care setting. Clinical Infectious Diseases. 2014;**58**:1219-1226

[30] Leon C, Ruiz-Santana S, Saavedra P, Galvan B, Blanco A, Castro C, et al. Usefulness of the "Candida score" for discriminating between Candida colonization and invasive candidiasis in non-neutropenic critically ill patients: A prospective multicenter study. Critical Care Medicine. 2009;**37**:1624-1633

[31] Gamaletsou MN, Walsh TJ, Zaoutis T, Pagoni M, Kotsopoulou M, Voulgarelis M, et al. A prospective, cohort, multicentre study of candidaemia in hospitalized adult patients with haematological malignancies. Clinical Microbiology and Infection. 2014;**20**:O50-O57

[32] Cesaro S, Tridello G, Blijlevens N, Ljungman P, Craddock C, Michallet M, et al. Incidence, risk factors and long-term outcome of acute leukemia patients with early candidemia after allogeneic stem cell transplantation. A study by the acute leukemia and infectious diseases working parties of EBMT. Clinical Infectious Diseases. 2018;**67**(4):564-572

[33] Pagano L, Dragonetti G, Cattaneo C, Marchesi F, Veggia B, Busca A, et al. Changes in the incidence of candidemia and related mortality in patients with hematologic malignancies in the last ten years. A SEIFEM 2015-B report. Haematologica. 2017;**102**:e407-ee10

[34] Raad I, Hanna H, Boktour M, Girgawy E, Danawi H, Mardani M, et al. Management of central venous catheters in patients with cancer and candidemia. Clinical Infectious Diseases. 2004;**38**: 1119-1127

[35] Wu PF, Liu WL, Hsieh MH, Hii IM, Lee YL, Lin YT, et al. Epidemiology and antifungal susceptibility of candidemia isolates of non-albicans Candida species from cancer patients. Emerging Microbes and Infections. 2017;**6**:e87

[36] Fernandez-Ruiz M, Puig-Asensio M, Guinea J, Almirante B, Padilla B, Almela M, et al. *Candida tropicalis* bloodstream infection: Incidence, risk factors and outcome in a population-based surveillance. The Journal of Infection. 2015;**71**:385-394

[37] Cortés JA, Cuervo SI, Hernandez LF, Potdevin G, Urdaneta AM. Ojo de buey en tomografia hepatica. Biomédica. 2004;**24**:7-12. DOI: 10.7705/biomedica.v24i1.1243

[38] Li D, Xia R, Zhang Q, Bai C, Li Z, Zhang P. Evaluation of candidemia in epidemiology and risk factors among cancer patients in a cancer center of China: An 8-year case-control study. BMC Infectious Diseases. 2017;**17**:536

[39] Tang HJ, Liu WL, Lin HL, Lai CC. Epidemiology and prognostic factors of candidemia in cancer patients. PLoS One. 2014;**9**:e99103

[40] Ortegon L, Puentes-Herrera M, Corrales IF, Cortes JA. Colonization and infection in the newborn infant: Does chlorhexidine play a role in infection prevention? Archivos Argentinos de Pediatría. 2017;**115**:65-70

[41] Chen J, Jiang Y, Wei B, Ding Y, Xu S, Qin P, et al. Epidemiology of and risk factors for neonatal candidemia at a tertiary care hospital in western China. BMC Infectious Diseases. 2016;**16**:700

[42] Benjamin DK Jr, Stoll BJ, Gantz MG, Walsh MC, Sanchez PJ, Das A, et al. Neonatal candidiasis: Epidemiology, risk factors, and clinical judgment. Pediatrics. 2010;**126**:e865-e873

[43] Benjamin DK Jr, Stoll BJ, Fanaroff AA, McDonald SA, Oh W, Higgins RD, et al. Neonatal candidiasis among extremely low birth weight infants: Risk factors, mortality rates, and

neurodevelopmental outcomes at 18 to 22 months. Pediatrics. 2006;**117**:84-92

[44] Orozco PA, Cortes JA, Parra CM. Colonization by yeasts in newborns and healthcare personnel in a neonatal intensive care unit at a university hospital in Bogota, Colombia. Revista Iberoamericana de Micología. 2009;**26**: 108-111

[45] Fu J, Wang X, Wei B, Jiang Y, Chen J. Risk factors and clinical analysis of candidemia in very-low-birth-weight neonates. American Journal of Infection Control. 2016;**44**:1321-1325

[46] Cleminson J, Austin N, McGuire W. Prophylactic systemic antifungal agents to prevent mortality and morbidity in very low birth weight infants. Cochrane Database of Systematic Reviews. 2015;**10**:CD003850

[47] van Schalkwyk E, Iyaloo S, Naicker SD, Maphanga TG, Mpembe RS, Zulu TG, et al. Large outbreaks of fungal and bacterial bloodstream infections in a neonatal unit, South Africa, 2012–2016. Emerging Infectious Diseases. 2018;**24**: 1204-1212

[48] Asmundsdottir LR, Erlendsdottir H, Haraldsson G, Guo H, Xu J, Gottfredsson M. Molecular epidemiology of candidemia: Evidence of clusters of smoldering nosocomial infections. Clinical Infectious Diseases. 2008;**47**:e17-e24

[49] Escribano P, Sanchez-Carrillo C, Munoz P, Bouza E, Guinea J. Reduction in percentage of clusters of *Candida albicans* and *Candida parapsilosis* causing candidemia in a general Hospital in Madrid, Spain. Journal of Clinical Microbiology. 2018;**56**(7): e00574-18

[50] Pappas PG, Kauffman CA, Andes DR, Clancy CJ, Marr KA, Ostrosky-Zeichner L, et al. Clinical practice guideline for the management of candidiasis: 2016 update by the Infectious Diseases Society of America. Clinical Infectious Diseases. 2016;**62**: e1-e50

[51] DiazGranados CA, Martinez A, Deaza C, Valderrama S. An outbreak of Candida spp. bloodstream infection in a tertiary care center in Bogota, Colombia. The Brazilian Journal of Infectious Diseases. 2008;**12**:390-394

[52] Li D, Li X, Xia R, Zhang W, Zheng S, Zhang Q, et al. Molecular surveillance of candidemia due to *Candida albicans* among cancer patients during 2009 to 2013 by microsatellite typing. Microbial Pathogenesis. 2015;**81**:28-32

[53] Bogomin F, Gago S, Oladele RO, Denning DW. Global and multi-national prevalence of fungal diseases—Estimate precision. Journal of Fungi. 2017;**3**:57

[54] Arendrup MC. Epidemiology of invasive candidiasis. Current Opinion in Critical Care. 2010;**16**:445-452

[55] Nucci M, Queiroz-Telles F, Alvarado-Matute T, Tiraboschi IN, Cortes J, Zurita J, et al. Epidemiology of candidemia in Latin America: A laboratory-based survey. PLoS One. 2013;**8**:e59373

[56] Lockhart SR, Iqbal N, Cleveland AA, Farley MM, Harrison LH, Bolden CB, et al. Species identification and antifungal susceptibility testing of Candida bloodstream isolates from population-based surveillance studies in two U.S. cities from 2008 to 2011. Journal of Clinical Microbiology. 2012; **50**:3435-3442

[57] Puig-Asensio M, Padilla B, Garnacho-Montero J, Zaragoza O, Aguado JM, Zaragoza R, et al. Epidemiology and predictive factors for early and late mortality in Candida bloodstream infections: A population-based surveillance in Spain. Clinical Microbiology and Infection. 2014;**20**: O245-O254

[58] Wang H, Xu YC, Hsueh PR. Epidemiology of candidemia and antifungal susceptibility in invasive Candida species in the Asia-Pacific region. Future Microbiology. 2016;**11**: 1461-1477

[59] Lortholary O, Renaudat C, Sitbon K, Madec Y, Denoeud-Ndam L, Wolff M, et al. Worrisome trends in incidence and mortality of candidemia in intensive care units (Paris area, 2002–2010). Intensive Care Medicine. 2014;**40**: 1303-1312

[60] Tan BH, Chakrabarti A, Li RY, Patel AK, Watcharananan SP, Liu Z, et al. Incidence and species distribution of candidaemia in Asia: A laboratory-based surveillance study. Clinical Microbiology and Infection. 2015;**21**: 946-953

[61] Lagrou K, Maertens J, Van Even E, Denning DW. Burden of serious fungal infections in Belgium. Mycoses. 2015;**58** (Supp. 5):1-5

[62] Arendrup MC, Fuursted K, Gahrn-Hansen B, Schonheyder HC, Knudsen JD, Jensen IM, et al. Semi-national surveillance of fungaemia in Denmark 2004–2006: Increasing incidence of fungaemia and numbers of isolates with reduced azole susceptibility. Clinical Microbiology and Infection. 2008;**14**: 487-494

[63] Poikonen E, Lyytikainen O, Anttila VJ, Koivula I, Lumio J, Kotilainen P, et al. Secular trend in candidemia and the use of fluconazole in Finland, 2004–2007. BMC Infectious Diseases. 2010;**10**:312

[64] Ruhnke M, Groll AH, Mayser P, Ullmann AJ, Mendling W, Hof H, et al. Estimated burden of fungal infections in Germany. Mycoses. 2015;**58**(Supp. 5): 22-28

[65] Sinko J, Sulyok M, Denning DW. Burden of serious fungal diseases in Hungary. Mycoses. 2015;**58**(Supp. 5): 29-33

[66] Dorgan E, Denning DW, McMullan R. Burden of fungal disease in Ireland. Journal of Medical Microbiology. 2015; **64**:423-426

[67] Nordoy I, Hesstvedt L, Torp Andersen C, Mylvaganam H, Kols NI, Falch BM, et al. An estimate of the burden of fungal disease in Norway. Journal of Fungi (Basel). 2018;**4**:E29

[68] Sabino R, Verissimo C, Brandao J, Martins C, Alves D, Pais C, et al. Serious fungal infections in Portugal. European Journal of Clinical Microbiology & Infectious Diseases. 2017;**36**:1345-1352

[69] Mares M, Moroti-Constantinescu VR, Denning DW. The burden of fungal diseases in Romania. Journal of Fungi (Basel). 2018;**4**:E31

[70] Klimko N, Kozlova Y, Khostelidi S, Shadrivova O, Borzova Y, Burygina E, et al. The burden of serious fungal diseases in Russia. Mycoses. 2015;**58** (Supp. 5):58-62

[71] Arsenijevic VA, Denning DW. Estimated burden of serious fungal diseases in Serbia. Journal of Fungi (Basel). 2018;**4**:E76

[72] Rodriguez-Tudela JL, Alastruey-Izquierdo A, Gago S, Cuenca-Estrella M, Leon C, Miro JM, et al. Burden of serious fungal infections in Spain. Clinical Microbiology and Infection. 2015;**21**: 183-189

[73] Ericsson J, Chryssanthou E, Klingspor L, Johansson AG, Ljungman P, Svensson E, et al. Candidaemia in Sweden: A nationwide prospective observational survey. Clinical Microbiology and Infection. 2013;**19**: E218-E221

[74] Osmanov A, Denning DW. Burden of serious fungal infections in Ukraine. Mycoses. 2015;**58**(Supp. 5):94-100

[75] Dufresne SF, Cole DC, Denning DW, Sheppard DC. Serious fungal infections in Canada. European Journal of Clinical Microbiology & Infectious Diseases. 2017;**36**:987-992

[76] Corzo-Leon DE, Armstrong-James D, Denning DW. Burden of serious fungal infections in Mexico. Mycoses. 2015;**58**(Supp. 5):34-44

[77] Cleveland AA, Harrison LH, Farley MM, Hollick R, Stein B, Chiller TM, et al. Declining incidence of candidemia and the shifting epidemiology of Candida resistance in two US metropolitan areas, 2008–2013: Results from population-based surveillance. PLoS One. 2015;**10**:e0120452

[78] Colombo AL, Nucci M, Park BJ, Nouer SA, Arthington-Skaggs B, da Matta DA, et al. Epidemiology of candidemia in Brazil: A nationwide sentinel surveillance of candidemia in eleven medical centers. Journal of Clinical Microbiology. 2006;**44**: 2816-2823

[79] Colombo AL, Guimaraes T, Sukienik T, Pasqualotto AC, Andreotti R, Queiroz-Telles F, et al. Prognostic factors and historical trends in the epidemiology of candidemia in critically ill patients: An analysis of five multicenter studies sequentially conducted over a 9-year period. Intensive Care Medicine. 2014;**40**: 1489-1498

[80] Riera FO, Caeiro JP, Denning DW. Burden of serious fungal infections in Argentina. Journal of Fungi (Basel). 2018;**4**:E151

[81] Giacomazzi J, Baethgen L, Carneiro LC, Millington MA, Denning DW, Colombo AL, et al. The burden of serious human fungal infections in Brazil. Mycoses. 2016;**59**:145-150

[82] Alvarez Duarte E, Denning DW. Serious fungal infections in Chile. European Journal of Clinical Microbiology & Infectious Diseases. 2017;**36**:983-986

[83] Alvarez-Moreno CA, Cortes JA, Denning DW. Burden of fungal infections in Colombia. Journal of Fungi (Basel). 2018;**4**

[84] Zurita J, Denning DW, Paz YMA, Solis MB, Arias LM. Serious fungal infections in Ecuador. European Journal of Clinical Microbiology & Infectious Diseases. 2017;**36**:975-981

[85] Medina N, Samayoa B, Lau-Bonilla D, Denning DW, Herrera R, Mercado D, et al. Burden of serious fungal infections in Guatemala. European Journal of Clinical Microbiology & Infectious Diseases. 2017;**36**:965-969

[86] Gugnani HC, Denning DW. Estimated burden of serious fungal infections in Jamaica by literature review and modelling. The West Indian Medical Journal. 2015;**64**:245-249

[87] Bustamante B, Denning DW, Campos PE. Serious fungal infections in Peru. European Journal of Clinical Microbiology & Infectious Diseases. 2017;**36**:943-948

[88] Denning DW, Gugnani HC. Burden of serious fungal infections in Trinidad and Tobago. Mycoses. 2015;**58**(Supp. 5): 80-84

[89] Macedo-Vinas M, Denning DW. Estimating the burden of serious fungal infections in Uruguay. Journal of Fungi (Basel). 2018;**4**:E37

[90] Gugnani HC, Denning DW, Rahim R, Sadat A, Belal M, Mahbub MS. Burden of serious fungal infections in Bangladesh. European Journal of Clinical Microbiology & Infectious Diseases. 2017;**36**:993-997

[91] Ben R, Denning DW. Estimating the burden of fungal diseases in Israel. The

Israel Medical Association Journal. 2015; **17**:374-379

[92] Wadi J, Denning DW. Burden of serious fungal infections in Jordan. Journal of Fungi (Basel). 2018;**4**:E15

[93] Kemaykin VM, Tabinbaev NB, Khudaibergenova MS, Olifirovich AA, Abdrakhmanova LM, Denning DW, et al. An estimate of severe and chronic fungal diseases in the Republic of Kazakhstan. Journal of Fungi (Basel). 2018;**4**:E34

[94] Huh K, Ha YE, Denning DW, Peck KR. Serious fungal infections in Korea. European Journal of Clinical Microbiology & Infectious Diseases. 2017;**36**:957-963

[95] Velayuthan RD, Samudi C, Lakhbeer Singh HK, Ng KP, Shankar EM, Denning DW. Estimation of the burden of serious human fungal infections in Malaysia. Journal of Fungi (Basel). 2018;**4**:E38

[96] Jabeen K, Farooqi J, Mirza S, Denning D, Zafar A. Serious fungal infections in Pakistan. European Journal of Clinical Microbiology & Infectious Diseases. 2017;**36**:949-956

[97] Batac MCR, Denning D. Serious fungal infections in the Philippines. European Journal of Clinical Microbiology & Infectious Diseases. 2017;**36**:937-941

[98] Taj-Aldeen SJ, Chandra P, Denning DW. Burden of fungal infections in Qatar. Mycoses. 2015;**58**(Supp. 5):51-57

[99] Chayakulkeeree M, Denning DW. Serious fungal infections in Thailand. European Journal of Clinical Microbiology & Infectious Diseases. 2017;**36**:931-935

[100] Tilavberdiev SA, Denning DW, Klimko NN. Serious fungal diseases in the Republic of Uzbekistan. European Journal of Clinical Microbiology & Infectious Diseases. 2017;**36**:925-929

[101] Xiao M, Sun ZY, Kang M, Guo DW, Liao K, Chen SC, et al. Five-year National Surveillance of invasive candidiasis: Species distribution and azole susceptibility from the China hospital invasive fungal surveillance net (CHIF-NET) study. Journal of Clinical Microbiology. 2018;**56**(7):e00577-18

[102] Chekiri-Talbi M, Denning DW. Burden of fungal infections in Algeria. European Journal of Clinical Microbiology & Infectious Diseases. 2017;**36**:999-1004

[103] Bamba S, Zida A, Sangare I, Cisse M, Denning DW, Hennequin C. Burden of severe fungal infections in Burkina Faso. Journal of Fungi (Basel). 2018;**4**: E35

[104] Mandengue CE, Denning DW. The burden of serious fungal infections in Cameroon. Journal of Fungi (Basel). 2018;**4**:E44

[105] Zaki SM, Denning DW. Serious fungal infections in Egypt. European Journal of Clinical Microbiology & Infectious Diseases. 2017;**36**:971-974

[106] Kalua K, Zimba B, Denning DW. Estimated burden of serious fungal infections in Malawi. Journal of Fungi (Basel). 2018;**4**:E61

[107] Sacarlal J, Denning DW. Estimated burden of serious fungal infections in Mozambique. Journal of Fungi (Basel). 2018;**4**:E75

[108] Faini D, Maokola W, Furrer H, Hatz C, Battegay M, Tanner M, et al. Burden of serious fungal infections in Tanzania. Mycoses. 2015;**58**(Supp. 5): 70-79

[109] Lortholary O, Desnos-Ollivier M, Sitbon K, Fontanet A, Bretagne S, Dromer F, et al. Recent exposure to

caspofungin or fluconazole influences the epidemiology of candidemia: A prospective multicenter study involving 2,441 patients. Antimicrobial Agents and Chemotherapy. 2011;**55**:532-538

[110] Maldonado NA, Cano LE, De Bedout C, Arbelaez CA, Roncancio G, Tabares AM, et al. Association of clinical and demographic factors in invasive candidiasis caused by fluconazole-resistant Candida species: A study in 15 hospitals, Medellin, Colombia 2010–2011. Diagnostic Microbiology and Infectious Disease. 2014;**79**: 280-286

[111] Garnacho-Montero J, Diaz-Martin A, Garcia-Cabrera E, Ruiz Perez de Pipaon M, Hernandez-Caballero C, Aznar-Martin J, et al. Risk factors for fluconazole-resistant candidemia. Antimicrobial Agents and Chemotherapy. 2010;**54**:3149-3154

[112] Mellinghoff SC, Panse J, Alakel N, Behre G, Buchheidt D, Christopeit M, et al. Primary prophylaxis of invasive fungal infections in patients with haematological malignancies: 2017 update of the recommendations of the Infectious Diseases Working Party (AGIHO) of the German Society for Haematology and Medical Oncology (DGHO). Annals of Hematology. 2018; **97**:197-207

[113] Leonart LP, Tonin FS, Ferreira VL, Penteado STS, Wiens A, Motta FA, et al. A network meta-analysis of primary prophylaxis for invasive fungal infection in haematological patients. Journal of Clinical Pharmacy and Therapeutics. 2017;**42**:530-538

[114] Satoh K, Makimura K, Hasumi Y, Nishiyama Y, Uchida K, Yamaguchi H. *Candida auris* sp. nov., a novel ascomycetous yeast isolated from the external ear canal of an inpatient in a Japanese hospital. Microbiology and Immunology. 2009;**53**:41-44

[115] Lee WG, Shin JH, Uh Y, Kang MG, Kim SH, Park KH, et al. First three reported cases of nosocomial fungemia caused by *Candida auris*. Journal of Clinical Microbiology. 2011;**49**: 3139-3142

[116] Chowdhary A, Sharma C, Duggal S, Agarwal K, Prakash A, Singh PK, et al. New clonal strain of *Candida auris*, Delhi, India. Emerging Infectious Diseases. 2013;**19**:1670-1673

[117] Magobo RE, Corcoran C, Seetharam S, Govender NP. *Candida auris*-associated candidemia, South Africa. Emerging Infectious Diseases. 2014;**20**:1250-1251

[118] Emara M, Ahmad S, Khan Z, Joseph L, Al-Obaid I, Purohit P, et al. *Candida auris* candidemia in Kuwait, 2014. Emerging Infectious Diseases. 2015;**21**:1091-1092

[119] Calvo B, Melo AS, Perozo-Mena A, Hernandez M, Francisco EC, Hagen F, et al. First report of *Candida auris* in America: Clinical and microbiological aspects of 18 episodes of candidemia. The Journal of Infection. 2016;**73**: 369-374

[120] McCarthy M. Hospital transmitted *Candida auris* infections confirmed in the US. BMJ. 2016;**355**:i5978

[121] Mizusawa M, Miller H, Green R, Lee R, Durante M, Perkins R, et al. Can multidrug-resistant *Candida auris* be reliably identified in clinical microbiology laboratories? Journal of Clinical Microbiology. 2017;**55**:638-640

[122] Arendrup MC, Prakash A, Meletiadis J, Sharma C, Chowdhary A. Comparison of EUCAST and CLSI reference microdilution MICs of eight antifungal compounds for *Candida auris* and associated tentative epidemiological cutoff values. Antimicrobial Agents and Chemotherapy. 2017;**61**(6): e00485-17

[123] Clancy CJ, Nguyen MH. Emergence of *Candida auris*: An international call to arms. Clinical Infectious Diseases. 2017;**64**:141-143

[124] Ruiz Gaitan AC, Moret A, Lopez Hontangas JL, Molina JM, Aleixandre Lopez AI, Cabezas AH, et al. Nosocomial fungemia by *Candida auris*: First four reported cases in continental Europe. Revista Iberoamericana de Micología. 2017;**34**:23-27

[125] Morales-Lopez SE, Parra-Giraldo CM, Ceballos-Garzon A, Martinez HP, Rodriguez GJ, Alvarez-Moreno CA, et al. Invasive infections with multidrug-resistant yeast *Candida auris*, Colombia. Emerging Infectious Diseases. 2017;**23**:162-164

[126] Borman AM, Szekely A, Johnson EM. Comparative pathogenicity of United Kingdom isolates of the emerging pathogen *Candida auris* and other key pathogenic Candida species. mSphere. 2016;**1**:e00189-16

[127] Lockhart SR, Etienne KA, Vallabhaneni S, Farooqi J, Chowdhary A, Govender NP, et al. Simultaneous emergence of multidrug-resistant *Candida auris* on 3 continents confirmed by whole-genome sequencing and epidemiological analyses. Clinical Infectious Diseases. 2017;**64**:134-140

[128] Gonzalez de Molina FJ, Leon C, Ruiz-Santana S, Saavedra P, Group CIS. Assessment of candidemia-attributable mortality in critically ill patients using propensity score matching analysis. Critical Care. 2012;**16**:R105

[129] Jia X, Li C, Cao J, Wu X, Zhang L. Clinical characteristics and predictors of mortality in patients with candidemia: A six-year retrospective study. European Journal of Clinical Microbiology & Infectious Diseases. 2018;**37**:1717-1724

[130] Cortes JA, Reyes P, Gomez CH, Cuervo SI, Rivas P, Casas CA, et al. Clinical and epidemiological characteristics and risk factors for mortality in patients with candidemia in hospitals from Bogota, Colombia. The Brazilian Journal of Infectious Diseases. 2014;**18**:631-637

[131] Barchiesi F, Orsetti E, Mazzanti S, Trave F, Salvi A, Nitti C, et al. Candidemia in the elderly: What does it change? PLoS One. 2017;**12**:e0176576

[132] Horn DL, Ostrosky-Zeichner L, Morris MI, Ullmann AJ, Wu C, Buell DN, et al. Factors related to survival and treatment success in invasive candidiasis or candidemia: A pooled analysis of two large, prospective, micafungin trials. European Journal of Clinical Microbiology & Infectious Diseases. 2010;**29**:223-229

[133] Bassetti M, Righi E, Ansaldi F, Merelli M, Scarparo C, Antonelli M, et al. A multicenter multinational study of abdominal candidiasis: Epidemiology, outcomes and predictors of mortality. Intensive Care Medicine. 2015;**41**: 1601-1610

[134] Raza A, Zafar W, Mahboob A, Nizammudin S, Rashid N, Sultan F. Clinical features and outcomes of Candidaemia in cancer patients: Results from Pakistan. The Journal of the Pakistan Medical Association. 2016;**66**: 584-589

[135] Cornely OA, Gachot B, Akan H, Bassetti M, Uzun O, Kibbler C, et al. Epidemiology and outcome of fungemia in a cancer Cohort of the Infectious Diseases Group (IDG) of the European Organization for Research and Treatment of Cancer (EORTC 65031). Clinical Infectious Diseases. 2015;**61**: 324-331

[136] Andes DR, Safdar N, Baddley JW, Playford G, Reboli AC, Rex JH, et al. Impact of treatment strategy on outcomes in patients with candidemia and other forms of invasive candidiasis:

A patient-level quantitative review of randomized trials. Clinical Infectious Diseases. 2012;**54**:1110-1122

[137] Lopez-Cortes LE, Almirante B, Cuenca-Estrella M, Garnacho-Montero J, Padilla B, Puig-Asensio M, et al. Empirical and targeted therapy of candidemia with fluconazole versus echinocandins: A propensity score-derived analysis of a population-based, multicentre prospective cohort. Clinical Microbiology and Infection. 2016; **22**(733):e1-e8

[138] Reboli AC, Rotstein C, Pappas PG, Chapman SW, Kett DH, Kumar D, et al. Anidulafungin versus fluconazole for invasive candidiasis. The New England Journal of Medicine. 2007;**356**: 2472-2482

Section 2

Environmental Mycology

Chapter 4

Fungal Growth and Aerosolization from Various Conditions and Materials

Jacob Mensah-Attipoe and Oluyemi Toyinbo

Abstract

Microorganisms, especially fungi, from damp indoor environments are known to be one of the main causes of degradation of indoor air quality and can pose serious health hazard to occupants because of the production of airborne particles. Particles produced during microbial growth include both living and non-living particles, which can be submicrometer in size. Individuals are exposed to fungi from various sources and in various conditions. The exposure may occur when the fungi grow in hidden areas and on materials that are in common areas and released under various conditions. The proliferation of fungi detected in a particular area depends on the species of fungi, the growth material and the conditions under which they are grown and released. Fungi aerosolized from any growth material include intact spores, which grow when deposited on favorable material surfaces and other fragments of the growth ranging from a few millimeters to micrometers in size. The types and amounts of intact spores and fragments aerosolized depend on factors such as air velocity blowing over the growth surface, the type of substrate, type of fungi, and relative humidity of the growth and the age of the fungal growth.

Keywords: fungi, growth, aerosolization, infections, exposure

1. Introduction

Fungal spores and fragments usually in the sub-micrometer size range can be released from contaminated materials into air, and if inhaled, may cause adverse health effects for people and animals [1–3]. There is increased interest in the role of aerosolized fungal spores and their submicrometer fragments in adverse effects considering the strong association between the numbers of fine particles and adverse health effects [4–7]. Furthermore, fungal exposures are receiving increasing attention as an occupational and public health problem; this is due to the high prevalence of fungal contamination in buildings. Dampness and moisture-related problems are the main sources of fungal contaminations [8, 9] in homes and other domestic dwellings [10] as well as schools [11].

Fungal spores and fragments are one of the most common classes of airborne biological aerosols in many indoor environments and they form part of the complex community of indoor biological agents [12–17]. Most of these particles are encountered in indoor environments where we spend about 90% of our time [18]. Because of this, it is important to determine the sources of these fungal spores and their fragments in such environments. Fungi from damp indoor environments are known to be one of the main causes of degradation of indoor air quality and can pose a serious health hazard to occupants [19, 20]. The submicrometer fragments are of utmost importance, because they tend to stay longer in air, and are easily inhaled. The smallest fragments (>0.1 μm) can deposit deep in the respiratory tract having the potential for causing adverse health effects [21–23]. Furthermore, the large surface area of the fragments relative to their mass may evoke high biological activity [22].

The high number of released fungal fragments in combination with their potential to deliver harmful antigens and mycotoxins to the alveolar region of the lung suggests the need for their characterization. Furthermore, the properties of spores and fragments released from fungal growth are dependent on the type of materials, the species of fungi, the cultivation time as well as the air volume passing over the growth. The characterization of fungal particles is important to help us understand the potential health effects associated with the exposure [21, 24]. Fungal spores are considered the most abundant fraction of these particles; they have an aerodynamic diameter (d_a) in the size range of 1–10 μm [25].

Indoor air, like outdoor air, has many sources of contaminants that affect health adversely. However, it is not clear which source is associated with the adverse health effects. As earlier explained, because we spend most of our time indoors, it is important to characterize fungal fragments based on their origin since this knowledge can improve our understanding of the potential adverse health effects associated with exposure to these particles.

It has been estimated that dampness and mold growth can be detected in most home as reviewed by Mudarri and Fisk [26] and have been associated with increases of 30–50% in several respiratory and asthma-related health outcomes [27]. Furthermore, approximately 8–18% of cases of acute bronchitis and 9–20% of respiratory infections are estimated to occur in environments contaminated with fungi [28].

The review of Samson et al. [29] claimed that floods, wet seasons, thermal modernization of residential buildings, air-conditioning systems, construction or material faults, and poor and improper ventilation are the major reasons for increase in the relative humidity and dampness of materials in the indoor environment. When moist conditions are prolonged in indoor environments, for example, when building materials stay damp for a long time, then the growth of microbes is promoted and there is an increased risk of microbial contamination [29–31]. In addition, certain characteristics of the home [32] as well as personal activities of its occupants [33] influence the microbial profile in indoor environments.

Generally, a wide range of fungal species may be encountered in the indoor air. For example, Zyska [34] surveyed the available literature and compiled a list of more than 200 fungal species present in air or growing on structural materials in indoor environments and therefore likely to contribute to the airborne fungal burden. Fungi in indoor environments can be inhaled and exposure via the airways is especially problematic. Furthermore, the presence of fungal particles has been linked to many diseases and symptoms among the occupants of moisture damage buildings [9, 19].

2. Indoor sources of fungi

There are several sources of fungal particles in the indoor environment. This includes fungal particles exclusively generated from indoor sources and those that infiltrate from the outdoor environment as shown in **Figure 1**.

Fungi found indoors may be from different sources. However, the majority (70–80%) of indoor fungal aerosol and fugal allergens (80%) are generated in the indoor environment [3]. In a study by Adams et al. [35], they observed that fungal

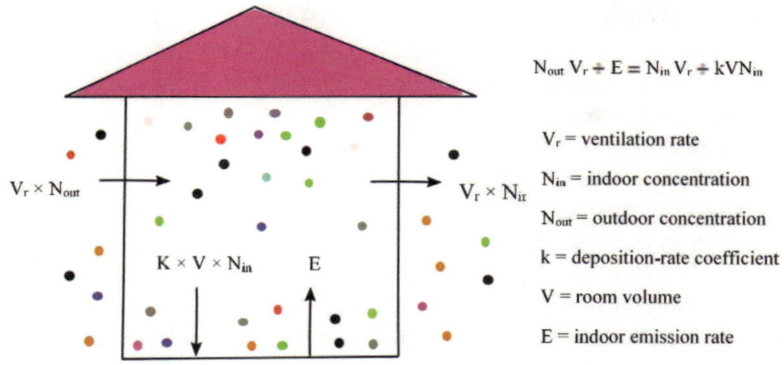

Figure 1.
Schematic diagram showing the sources of fungal particles in the indoor environment [3]. Reproduced with permission from Yamamoto et al.

composition indoor was related to dispersal from the outdoor environment and are passively collected by indoor surfaces, although they rarely grow on the surfaces.

In addition to the above, the basic characteristics and parts of a building can also affect the emergence of fungi. Different researches including Despot and Klarić [36] and Toyinbo et al. [37] have associated buildings with basements with the emergence of indoor mold. This may be due to the high humidity and cold temperature in the building basement. The high humidity and/moisture content may occur from leaky pipes or cracks in the basement walls that allow ground water to penetrate the basement. Another source of moisture in the basement is flooding which makes water to move down to the basement and usually dry at a slow rate due to lack of adequate ventilation. This creates a favorable condition for fungal growth. The kitchen and bathroom sections of a building may also encourage the growth of fungi since these places have a high moisture content and substrates [38].

Outdoor generated indoor fungi enter a building through the ventilation system. This can be a mechanical ventilation system without adequate air filter for pollutants or through a naturally ventilated building with open windows and doors where outdoor to indoor ratio of pollutants can be close to unity. A ventilation system can also be a reservoir for indoor fungi especially when the ducts and filters are dirty with dust that serves as a substrate for fungi growth [39]. A DNA-based analysis of air handling unit filters by Luhung et al. [40] shows diverse genera of fungi, which includes *Cladosporium, Aspergillus* and *Lentinus.* Oil residues in ventilation ducts can also trap dusts and serves as a source of nutrients for fungal growth that can be transferred indoor through the ventilation system [39].

3. Health effects of fungi in indoor environment

The health effects associated with fungal exposures may be caused by the fungi themselves, fungal mycotoxins, and fungal cell wall components or metabolically produced volatile compounds. The health effects can be categorized into three groups: (1) infections, which are caused mostly by the viable cells; (2) allergic reactions, which are usually caused by both viable and non-viable cells and components of the cell wall of the fungi if they carry antigens and (3) toxic responses, usually in response to the mycotoxins produced by the fungi.

Exposure to fungal particles has been linked to a range of adverse health effects [41]. For example, exposure to fungi has been associated with the onset of asthma in both infants and adults [42–47].

There is convincing data in the literature suggesting an association between moisture damage in a building and the incidence of diseases such as new asthma cases, current asthma, respiratory infections, cough, allergic rhinitis, eczema and bronchitis [2, 42, 43, 46–49]. In contrast, quantitative assessments have not detected any consistent associations between fungal measurements and adverse health effects. Nevertheless, limited or sufficient associations have been documented between the fungal concentration in dust by qPCR, cultured airborne fungi sampled from indoor air as well as several microbial compounds such as ergosterol, endotoxins and beta-glucans in dust and adverse health effects [50–53]. There is credible scientific evidence to support the association between moisture damage, visible fungal growth measured indoors and adverse health effects. The World Health Organization (WHO) has stated that approximately 25% of residents in social housing stocks are prone to experience elevated health risks associated with their exposure to indoor molds.

4. Fungi and fungal growth

Fungi are eukaryotic organisms that lack chlorophyll and obtain their nutrients from the growth media by the use of enzymes that they secrete. On the other hand, molds are filamentous fungi that grow with branched multi-cellular filamentous structures called mycelium [54]. In general, fungi are characterized by a visible vegetative body or a colony composed of a network of threadlike filaments which infiltrate the materials on which they feed. Fungi are usually saprophytic in nature; thus, they obtain nutrients from dead organic matter provided there is sufficient moisture. They can live off many of the materials present in the indoor environment such as wood, cellulose, insulations, wallpapers, glue and everyday dust and dirt [55–57]. Thus, fungi have the remarkable capability to degrade almost all natural and man-made materials [15, 58, 59] especially if they are hygroscopic [10, 60]. Fungi obtain nutrients by releasing extracellular enzymes and acids that break down the materials prior to their absorption. In the process, particles, including microbial degraded materials as well as gases, especially microbial volatile organic compounds (MVOCs), are released into the environment [61].

The MVOCs may form sub-micrometer particles through a process of secondary aerosol formation [61, 62]. These sub-micrometer particles have been shown to be aerosolized into the indoor environment following exposure to the effects of airflows and vibration [62, 63] **Figure 2**.

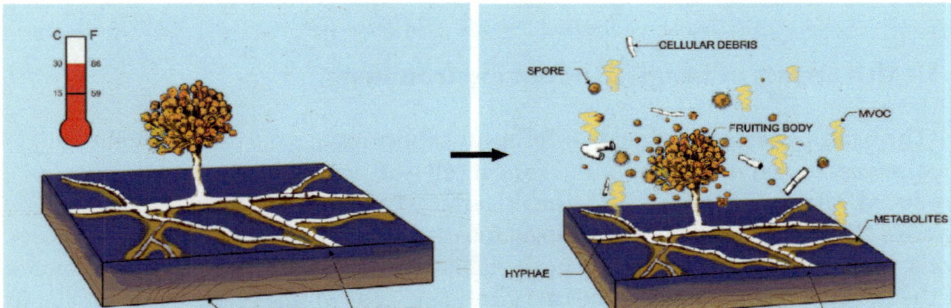

Figure 2.
Schematic diagram showing the growth of fungi on a material surface with the subsequent release of particles of the fungal growth [64]. Reproduced with permission from Morse and acker.

5. Conditions that promote fungal growth indoors

5.1 Material characteristics

Distinct characteristics of the growth material can play an important role in the creation and accumulation of moisture which eventually lead to mold growth on their surfaces [65, 66]. For example, when building are constructed with very good insulations in order to reduce heat loss and improve thermal performance, the several layers of insulation prevent easy movement of air in and through the building materials leading to accumulation of moisture within the building materials as well as the building. Consequently, the building becomes a microbiological reservoir and a contributor to the microbial exposure due to their ability to absorb and accumulate moisture [67].

Due to the heterogeneous nature of new buildings, there are varieties of materials that serve as micro-niches, that is, they have a favorable temperature, water activity (a_w) and relative humidity (RH). For example, the surfaces of affected building materials (such as concrete and ceramic tiles in moist walls, ceiling tiles, dust laden wooden furniture) create specific niches suitable for the growth of microorganisms including bacteria and fungi. As expected, the climate within the building varies from one part of the indoor environment to the next. Thus, fungal growth would also be predicted to vary with the microclimate created. Moisture damage and dampness in buildings often affect a variety of structural components of building materials, leading to a deterioration of the indoor air quality.

5.2 Water, nutrients and temperature requirements

Water-damaged building materials, particularly those rich in organic matter, can support microbial growth if they remain wet for a prolonged period of time [55, 59]. Under certain required conditions such as temperature, nutrient and pH conditions, microbial growth can occur within an hour [24]. Nonetheless, the principal limiting factor is the availability of moisture [55, 68]. It has been established that the lowest RH of a material at which fungi can grow is in a range around 75–80%, which corresponds to a water activity (a_w) of 0.75–80 [55, 69, 70]. The moisture of the substrate that is available to the fungi for growth is the so-called free water and this amount is influenced by the relative humidity of the surrounding air. This does not include bound water that is a component of the chemistry of the substrate [24]. Moisture sources for fungal growth on materials indoors may be internal or external with moisture movement into and through building cavities by convection, gravity or capillary action.

Pasanen et al. [71] found that relative humidity values of 70–90% are required if there is to be fungal growth on building materials. Furthermore, the relative humidity required for growth depends on the particular material and the fungal species involved. Since most materials are porous in nature, adsorption of water into the materials first occurs via the pores before the material surface and become available to the microbes. Thus, porous materials support fungal growth when their RH is higher than 80% [68]. These conditions influence the extent of colonization and the types of fungi that will be present, since any changes in moisture availability will change also the composition of the microbial species present in that environment. For example, certain species of *Penicillium, Erotium* and *Aspergillus* grow in relatively dry environments with RH between 75 and 85% (e.g., in settled house dust on material surfaces with a relatively low RH). As RH increases, different species such as *Basidiomycetes* and *Eratonium* begin to grow, requiring continuously wet substrates such as soaked wallboard with RH range of 80–90%, while others like *Fusarium, Cladosporium* and *Stachybotrys* only grow at RH exceeding 90% [29, 70–73].

In addition to humidity and water, fungi need adequate nutrition and temperatures to grow. The availability of nutrients depends on the composition of the building material. Building materials like wood and ceiling tiles are organic in nature; they contain complex polymers like starch, cellulose and lignin. These components are broken down by the extracellular enzymes of the fungi into simple sugars, amino acids and other simple nutrients [74, 75]. As fungi can utilize many complex polymers, a wide range of materials can act as nutrient sources.

Fungi can grow over a wide temperature range (5–39°C), [76]. However, at low temperatures (0–5°C), the fungal metabolic activities necessary for growth are slowed down, rendering the fungi dormant until an optimum temperature is reached [77]. At a higher temperature (34–36°C) the metabolic reaction rates increase and at temperatures above 46°C, the fungi become stressed and die [78]. This is because most of the activities of the fungi are dependent on DNA and enzymes. Due to the above, the concentration of fungi is usually high during the summer season as compared to winter season [79].

5.3 Types of building materials

Fungal growth on building materials is dependent on the chemical composition of the materials [58]. The most susceptible materials to microbial growth and biodegradation are those with a natural organic composition, for example, wood and paper. These materials contain starch, cellulose and hemicellulose, pectin and lignin [74, 80, 81]. Based on these components, a wide variety of materials are potentially suitable for supporting fungal growth [15, 58, 59].

Buildings contain a wide variety of materials that affect the germination and growth rate of fungi [82]. Thus, each material serves as a niche for a specific microorganism, depending on the composition of the material, water activity and nutrient content [58, 83]. These properties of the building materials determine the diversity and extent of growth of the microbes [84, 85].

Wood remains the most extensively used material in buildings [81, 86]. Wood is able to absorb and retain water and moisture from both standing water and the environment [81, 87]. This characteristic in addition to the high nitrogen-bound compounds and low molecular carbohydrates that are transferred to the wood surface during processing mean that wood is very susceptible to fungal growth [87]. For example, a study by Meklin et al. [88] found school constructed with wood to have a higher concentration of fungi (5–950 cfu/m^3) than those constructed with concrete (<2–5 to 500 cfu/m^3). Although concrete is also hygroscopic, it has a low moisture permeability which reduces its rate of degradation and it contains very little or no nutrient for fungi growth [89]. Fungal species commonly found on moisture-damaged wood include *Aspergillus versicolor, Penicillium brevicompactum*, [81, 84, 85].

Gypsum board, on the other hand, is mostly used as the inner wall liners in buildings [90]. The paper liners used to reinforce the gypsum core makes gypsum board susceptible to fungal growth. Since the inner core (gypsum) is able to retain water and make it available to the surface paper lining, there can be a prolonged presence of water and moisture required to sustain fungal growth [10]. While the inner core (gypsum) may not be susceptible to fungal growth, the glue and paper serve as good media due to their organic nature [91]. The fungal species routinely found on gypsum board are the cellulolytic *Stachybotrys chartarum* [70] and *Cladosporium cladosporioides* [91].

Plastic materials are also becoming a common material used in buildings, as either sheets or pipes. As sheets, they are used as material envelopes, which insulate the building. Though plastics are known to be resistant to microbial attack because microbes do not possess any enzymes capable of degrading synthetic polymers [92], the addition of plasticizers can make the plastics susceptible to microbial growth [93]. These plasticizers are commonly organic acid esters such as dioctylphthalates (DOP) and dioctyladipate (DOA) which are added to the polyvinyl chloride (PVC) to modify the polymer's physical or mechanical properties [93].

Glass fibers used in insulation materials do not support fungal growth. However, the glue used as binders does contain nutrients that may promote fungal growth [90] since these glues can be synthetic or plant-based. For example, the urea-based derivatives, polyurethanes, which are used as binders, are known to support fungal growth [94]. Plant-based binders are also used in binding certain building materials such as plywood, and ceiling tiles and may contain nutrients suitable to allow fungal growth.

5.4 Contamination or soiling

All materials, both organic and inorganic, are able to sustain fungal life especially when the materials have dust, dirt or other deposits on their surface which represent sources of carbon and nitrogen [56, 57]. Dust is known to contain microorganisms, debris and other animal or insect parts that serve as nutrients for fungal growth [95]. Thus, more growth is observed on materials with dust on their surfaces compared to those without dust [56, 96]. Furthermore, settled dust or soil alters the water absorbing and retentive characteristics of the material surface, making the material surface continually moist, conditions in which fungi thrive [10]. Dust absorbs water from the atmosphere. It has been shown that dust competes with the material surface for moisture, with the dust holding more water due to its more hygroscopic nature. Therefore, dust may promote fungal growth even on materials that naturally would not support microbial growth [56, 57]. It is therefore important for indoor surfaces to be continually cleaned to avoid fungal growth and any health effect associated with it.

6. Aerosolization of fungal spores and fragments

Forces such as turbulence, temperature, air velocity, vibration and zone of convection are usually associated with the release of fungal spores and hyphae from fungal colonies. In addition, factors such as the maturity of the colony, changes in temperature, relative humidity over the culture surface, light periods, nutritional composition of the substrate and the specific fungal species will determine the frequency and the number of spores that will be liberated and transported into the air at any given time. Furthermore, the dispersal of the fungal particles depends upon their size, shape, roughness, density, electrostatic charge, air movement and activities that influence the circulation of the air [24].

Release of fungal particles usually occurs by two mechanisms; active and passive release [68]. Active release refers to an adaptive type of particle aerosolization, via forces arising inside the fungi attributable to a burst of energy by a mechanism known as osmotic pressure and surface tension discharge [97]. Passive release occurs by energy originating from outside the fungi, such as mechanical disturbances of the fungal colonies by mechanical handling, vibration or air currents. The latter forces can also cause secondary release of settled spores from surfaces. Activities that have been shown to increase fungal spore concentrations in indoor air include daily activities such as vacuuming, sweeping, walking etc. [98–103].

During fungal growth and sporulation, as well as when the culture is in a dormant phase, spores and bioactive agent containing fragments are released into the indoor environment [21, 61, 104–107]. As mentioned earlier, hyphal fragments are of high importance since they make up about 6–56% of the total fungal particles based on microscopic sample analysis [108, 109]. Aerosolized fungal particles in chamber studies have shown that fungal fragments are released at levels up to 514 times higher than spores [21, 61, 106, 107, 110]. In other studies, Li and Kendrick [111] used microscopic counting and found that hyphal fragments accounted for only 6.3% of the total number of fungal particles in indoor environments. In addition, by applying a biomass determination, Adhikari et al. [112] detected lower amounts of β-N-acetylhexosaminidase (NAHA) enzyme in fungal fragments <1 μm compared to spores >1.8 μm.

Though both types of particles (spores and fragments) released from the fungal cultures during aerosolization are potentially harmful, the fragments are of greater importance since they tend to suspend longer in air than the spores [61, 62, 106, 107, 113]. They also have a tendency to penetrate deep into alveolar regions of the respiratory tract when inhaled [21, 114]. Cho et al. [21] have used a computer-based model to assess the deposition of spores and fragments of *A. versicolor* and *S. chartarum* in the respiratory tract. For both fungi, they found that the vast majority, 65–90%, of inhaled fungal spores deposited in the nasal and extra thoracic regions while only 3–15 and 2–5% of the spores deposited in the alveoli-interstitial and bronchial-bronchiolar regions, respectively. They also demonstrated that about 60% of fungal fragments deposited in the alveoli-interstitial region with 14–15% being trapped in the nasal and extrathoracic regions. It can therefore be deduced from the above modeling analysis that the different deposition efficiencies could have consequences on the potential adverse health effects induced by inhaled fungal particles of different sizes.

Fungal fragments have been shown to contain antigens [61, 62], allergens [5, 115, 116], mycotoxins [23, 117], and (1 → 3)-β-D-glucans [23, 52]. Their size in relation to their numbers and their biological properties all contribute to their potential to evoke adverse health effects. It is known from atmospheric studies investigating the adverse health effects of ultrafine particles that it is the number concentration rather than mass concentration which is important [118, 119].

Different fungal species have characteristic structures and thus behave differently when they become airborne. In addition, the growth substrate providing the nutrients for the fungi may also affect the properties of the spores and fragments and could contribute to fragments released from the biodegradation of the substrate itself during fungal metabolism. The amount of fungal particles released may also depend on the type of substrate and the conditions under which the fungi were grown. It is very important to evaluate spore properties under a variety of conditions in order to gain insights into the contribution these factors have on the adverse health effects produced by these particles.

7. Aerosolization and characterization of fungal spores and fragments

One of the ways fungal particles are characterized is by their properties when they are released from contaminated materials. The particles released are affected by the growth substrate, fungal species, age of the culture and air velocity to which the cultures had been exposed [120]. The same factors affected the fragment/spore (F/S) ratios [121].

Biological particles are usually distinguished from non-biological particles by their ability to fluoresce when excited with photons at a certain wavelength. The fluorescence property is based on molecules such as tryptophan, tyrosine, or phenylalanine, reduced nicotinamide adenine dinucleotide (NADH), and nicotinamide adenine dinucleotide phosphate (NADPH) as well as riboflavins, flavin adenine dinucleotide (FADH) and flavin mononucleotide (FMN). Depending on the conditions under which the fungi grow, differences in fluorescence properties are observed. For example, spores obtained from cultures on building materials, such as, gypsum board, have been shown to have lower fluorescent properties than spores from agar. This indicates that cultures growing on nutrient poor substrates contain less compounds capable of fluorescence. Studies by Agranovski et al. [121] and Kanaani et al. [122] measuring fungal amounts from agar using fluorescence measuring devices in laboratory settings resulted in good detection efficiency of the instruments. However, the use of fluorescence properties may underestimate the concentration of fungal particles due to influences of nutrient availability on the growth of the fungi.

The type of species also affects the fluorescence properties. For example, lower fluorescent particle fraction (FPF) values have been observed for *C. cladosporioides* compared to *A. versicolor* and *P. brevicompactum* [120, 123]. The structure of the spore plays a major role in allowing devices to measure fluorescence properties. *C. cladosporioides* has a dark-skinned coating preventing impinging photons from penetrating to reach the exterior pigments to excite fluorescence from internal fluorescence. It can be deduced that *C. cladosporioides* concentrations may be underestimated in field measurements.

In recent study by Mensah-Attipoe et al. [121] and Afanou et al. [104], they observed that *A. versicolor* produced a higher F/S-ratio compared to *C. cladosporioides* and *P. brevicompactum*. The increased sub-micrometer fragments from *A. versicolor* can be attributed to the outer-wall spines, which are easily sheared away during sampling.

Studies have shown that the type of material and nutrient affects how much particles are released [120, 121]. For example, the fragment/spore ratio (F/S) for agar was higher compared to wood and gypsum board. Seo et al. [124] observed a higher F/S ratio for *A. versicolor* cultivated on agar than on gypsum board and ceiling tiles. Generally, higher concentrations of fungal particles are aerosolized from dry surfaces with low moisture contents than wet surfaces with high humidity [62]. Agar may have a different moisture content and moisture dynamics during the fungal growth than wood and gypsum board. During growth, the moisture content becomes reduced [23] and it is possible that agar loses more moisture than wood and gypsum. Therefore, fungal growth on agar undergoes desiccation stress and releases more fragment particles than when it grows on wood and gypsum board.

It has been observed that fragment/spore ratio (F/S) increases with increasing age of the culture. Moisture content of wood and gypsum increases with incubation time. Therefore, before aerosolization can yield enough particles, the material must be dried. With differences in the absorption and retention of moisture by the various materials, fungal biomass is also affected and hence affects the release dynamics of fungal particles from the material surfaces. Seo et al. [124] demonstrated that F/S increased with age. They attributed the increase in particle release from older cultures to changes in fungal biomass and moisture content. Dryness on the surface of the culture increases the aerosolization of fungal particles by reducing the adhesion forces between the fungal structures and making these structures more brittle [124]. Therefore, it has been concluded that with time, fungal growth in buildings may increase the contribution of sub-micrometer-sized fungal fragments to the overall mold exposure [124]. Spores aerosolized from older cultures displayed lower fluorescence than younger cultures. Kanaani et al. [125] reported a decrease in fluorescence emitted by *Penicillium* and *Aspergillus* from 2 days to 21 days. They suggested that fluorescent intensity of biomolecules such as nicotinamide-adenine dinucleotide phosphate NAD(P)H and surrogates of metabolic function such as riboflavin found in fungal spores may vary according to the environmental conditions under which the fungal colonies are growing and also on their concentration at a particular point in time. The decrease in fluorescence with age could also be due to changes in the fluorescent compounds as the culture ages.

Concentration of fungal spores and fragments has been shown to increase with increasing air velocity, but the F/S ratios decreased with increase in air velocity. A decrease in fluorescence per spore was observed when the air velocity was increased. It is also possible that as larger particles are carried along with the increased air currents in the sampling lines, they impact on the sides of the walls resulting in the breakage; as posited by Afanou et al. [104, 105].

Fragments have been proposed to be secondary organic aerosols formed from MVOCs released from fungal growths (secondary formation of aerosol particles) [61]. If fragment particles are formed by this mechanism in the presence of ozone, the concentration of fragments should decrease with higher flow rates due to their increased dilution. However, the opposite was observed by Mensah-Attipoe et al. [121], meaning that secondary aerosol formation may not be a relevant process for origin of fungal fragments. Instead, fragments are mainly formed through mechanical processes. It has been shown that fungal fragments are aerosolized at low air velocity [61]. Studies by Mensah-Attipoe et al. [121] show that fragments and spore concentrations increased with greater air velocities, however, the spore concentration increased more than the fragment concentration. This explains the decrease in F/S ratio when the air velocity is increased. A decrease in fluorescence in response to the increase in air velocity has been postulated to be due to a decrease in relative humidity of the culture causing desiccation stress to the fungal spores [125]. In addition, due to the increased air velocity, larger fungal hyphae are aerosolized together with spores due to increased stress and desiccation of the colony. The desiccation stress and decrease in fluorescence induced by increased air velocity has been attributed to a loss of spore viability [125].

8. Conclusions

The type of building material and fungal species affect the amount of growth measured on the contaminated surfaces. In addition, these factors together with air velocity and age of the culture affect the properties of the fungal particles aerosolized from fungal contaminated surfaces. The nutritional value, chemical composition and moisture requirements as well as sources of external nutrients potentially affect fungal growth.

Fluorescence property of the particles which is sometimes attributed to their viability decreases when fungi are grown on poor nutrient substrates, released from older cultures and released in the presence of high air velocities. Since a building has many different materials in its structure and varying airflows passing over different ages of the growths at any point in time, it is concluded that fungal viability and their ability to cause infections may vary under different conditions.

F/S ratios decrease with increasing air velocity while spore concentration increase. This suggests that the conditions under which individuals are exposed to fungal particles may be different. A fraction of the fragments could be derived from building materials due to biodegradation of substrates when they are subjected to fungal metabolism. Fragments aerosolized from building materials could represent a potential health hazard depending on the composition of the material.

Author details

Jacob Mensah-Attipoe* and Oluyemi Toyinbo
Department of Environmental and Biological Sciences, University of Eastern Finland, Kuopio, Finland

*Address all correspondence to: jacob.mensah-attipoe@uef.fi

References

[1] Chew GL, Rogers C, Burge HA, Muilenberg ML, Gold DR. Dustborne and airborne fungal propagules represent a different spectrum of fungi with differing relations to home characteristics. Allergy. 2003;**58**(1):13-20

[2] Mendell MJ, Mirer AG, Cheung K, Tong M, Douwes J. Respiratory and allergic health effects of dampness, mold, and dampness-related agents: A review of the epidemiologic evidence. Environmental Health Perspectives. 2011;**119**(6):748-756

[3] Yamamoto N, Hospodsky D, Dannemiller KC, Nazaroff WW, Peccia J. Indoor emissions as a primary source of airborne allergenic fungal particles in classrooms. Environmental Science & Technology. 2015;**49**(8):5098-5106

[4] Gold DR et al. Ambient pollution and heart rate variability. Circulation. 2000;**101**(11):1267-1273

[5] Green BJ, Tovey ER, Sercombe JK, Blachere FM, Beezhold DH, Schmechel D. Airborne fungal fragments and allergenicity. Medical Mycology. 2006;**44**(sup 1):245-255

[6] Magari SR, Hauser R, Schwartz J, Williams PL, Smith TJ, Christiani DC. Association of heart rate variability with occupational and environmental exposure to particulate air pollution. Circulation. 2001;**104**(9):986-991

[7] Pekkanen J et al. Particulate air pollution and risk of ST-segment depression during repeated submaximal exercise tests among subjects with coronary heart disease: The exposure and risk assessment for fine and ultrafine particles in ambient air (ULTRA) study. Circulation. 2002;**106**(8):933-938

[8] Institute of Medicine (IOM). Committee on damp indoor spaces and health. In: Damp Indoor Spaces and Health. Washington, D.C.: National Academies Press; 2004

[9] Heseltine E, Rosen J. WHO Guidelines for Indoor Air Quality: Dampness and Mould. Europe: WHO Regional Office; 2009

[10] Flannigan B, Samson RA, Miller JD, editors. Microorganisms in indoor air. In: Microorganisms in Home and Indoor Work Environments: Diversity, Health Impacts, Investigation and Control. London: Taylor & Francis; 2001. pp. 17-31

[11] Norback D et al. Mould and dampness in dwelling places, and onset of asthma: The population-based cohort ECRHS. Occupational and Environmental Medicine. 2013;**70**(5):325-331

[12] Bauer H et al. Significant contributions of fungal spores to the organic carbon and to the aerosol mass balance of the urban atmospheric aerosol. Atmospheric Environment. 2008;**42**(22):5542-5549

[13] Dacarro C, Picco AM, Grisoli P, Rodolfi M. Determination of aerial microbiological contamination in scholastic sports environments. Journal of Applied Microbiology. 2003;**95**(5):904-912

[14] Elbert W, Taylor PE, Andreae MO, Pöschl U. Contribution of fungi to primary biogenic aerosols in the atmosphere: Wet and dry discharged spores, carbohydrates, and inorganic ions. Atmospheric Chemistry and Physics. 2007;**7**(17):4569-4588

[15] Nevalainen A, Seuri M. Of microbes and men. Indoor Air. 2005;**15**(Suppl 9):58-64

[16] Reponen T, Willeke K, Grinshpun S, Nevalainen A. Biological particle sampling. In: Kulkarni P, Baron P, Willeke K, editors. Aerosol Measurement, Principles,

Techniques, and Applications. 3rd ed. Hoboken, NJ: John Wiley & Johns, Inc.; 2011. pp. 549-570

[17] Womiloju TO, Miller JD, Mayer PM, Brook JR. Methods to determine the biological composition of particulate matter collected from outdoor air. Atmospheric Environment. 2003;**37**(31):4335-4344

[18] Esmen NA. The status of indoor air pollution. Environmental Health Perspectives. 1985;**62**:259

[19] Gutarowska B, Piotrowska M. Methods of mycological analysis in buildings. Building and Environment. 2007;**42**(4):1843-1850

[20] Madsen AM et al. Generation and characterization of indoor fungal aerosols for inhalation studies. Applied and Environmental Microbiology. 2016;**82**:2479-2493. AEM-04063

[21] Cho S-H, Seo S-C, Schmechel D, Grinshpun SA, Reponen T. Aerodynamic characteristics and respiratory deposition of fungal fragments. Atmospheric Environment. 2005;**39**(30):5454-5465

[22] Frankel M, Hansen EW, Madsen AM.Effect of relative humidity on the aerosolization and total inflammatory potential of fungal particles from dust-inoculated gypsum boards. Indoor Air. 2014;**24**(1):16-28

[23] Seo SC, Reponen T, Levin L, Borchelt T, Grinshpun SA. Aerosolization of particulate (1–>3)-beta-D-glucan from moldy materials. Applied and Environmental Microbiology. 2008;**74**(3):585-593

[24] McGinnis MR. Indoor mould development and dispersal. Medical Mycology. 2007;**45**(1):1-9

[25] Glikson M, Rutherford S, Simpson RW, Mitchell CA, Yago A. Microscopic and submicron components of atmospheric particulate matter during high asthma periods in Brisbane, Queensland, Australia. Atmospheric Environment. 1995;**29**(4):549-562

[26] Mudarri D, Fisk WJ. Public health and economic impact of dampness and mold. Indoor Air. 2007;**17**(3):226-235

[27] Fisk WJ, Lei-Gomez Q, Mendell MJ. Meta-analyses of the associations of respiratory health effects with dampness and mold in homes. Indoor Air. 2007;**17**(4):284-296

[28] Fisk WJ, Eliseeva EA, Mendell MJ. Association of residential dampness and mold with respiratory tract infections and bronchitis: A meta-analysis. Environmental Health: Global Access Sci. Sour. 2010;**9**:72

[29] Samson RA, Houbraken J, Thrane U, Frisvad JC, Andersen B. Food and Indoor Fungi. CBS laboratory manual series 2. Utrecht: CBS-KNAW Fungal Biodiversity Centre; 2010

[30] Piñar G, Sterflinger K. Microbes and building materials. In: Build. Mater. Prop. Perform. New York: Appl. Nov. Publ; 2009. pp. 163-188

[31] Sterflinger K. Fungi: Their role in deterioration of cultural heritage. Fungal Biology Reviews. 2010;**24**(1):47-55

[32] Sordillo JE, Alwis UK, Hoffman E, Gold DR, Milton DK. Home characteristics as predictors of bacterial and fungal microbial biomarkers in house dust. Environmental Health Perspectives. 2010;**119**(2):189-195

[33] Dunn RR, Fierer N, Henley JB, Leff JW, Menninger HL. Home life: Factors structuring the bacterial diversity found within and between homes. PLoS ONE. 2013;**8**(5):e64133

[34] Zyska B. Fungi in indoor air in European countries. Mikologia Lekarska. 2001;**8**(3/4):127-140

[35] Adams RI, Miletto M, Taylor JW, Bruns TD. The diversity and distribution of fungi on residential surfaces. PLoS One. 2013;**8**(11):e78866

[36] Despot DJ, Klarić MŠ. A year-round investigation of indoor airborne fungi in Croatia. Archives of Industrial Hygiene and Toxicology. 2014;**65**(2):209-218

[37] Toyinbo O, Matilainen M, Turunen M, Putus T, Shaughnessy R, Haverinen-Shaughnessy U. Modeling associations between principals' reported indoor environmental quality and students' self-reported respiratory health outcomes using GLMM and ZIP models. International Journal of Environmental Research and Public Health. 2016;**13**(4):385

[38] Mentese S, Arisoy M, Rad AY, Güllü G. Bacteria and fungi levels in various indoor and outdoor environments in Ankara, Turkey. Clean—Soil, Air, Water. 2009;**37**(6):487-493

[39] Khan AAH, Karuppayil SM. Fungal pollution of indoor environments and its management. Saudi Journal of Biological Sciences. 2012;**19**(4):405

[40] Luhung I, Wu Y, Xu S, Yamamoto N, Chang VW-C, Nazaroff WW. DNA accumulation on ventilation system filters in university buildings in Singapore. PLoS One. 2017;**12**(10):e0186295

[41] Douwes J, Thorne P, Pearce N, Heederik D. Bioaerosol health effects and exposure assessment: Progress and prospects. The Annals of Occupational Hygiene. 2003;**47**(3):187-200

[42] Bornehag C-G et al. Dampness in buildings and health. Indoor Air. 2001;**11**(2):72-86

[43] Bornehag C-G et al. Dampness in buildings as a risk factor for health effects, EUROEXPO: A multidisciplinary review of the literature (1998-2000) on dampness and mite exposure in buildings and health effects. Indoor Air. 2004;**14**(4):243-257

[44] Johanning E. Indoor moisture and mold-related health problems. European Annals of Allergy and Clinical Immunology. 2004;**36**(5):182-185

[45] Johanning E, Auger P, Morey PR, Yang CS, Olmsted E. Review of health hazards and prevention measures for response and recovery workers and volunteers after natural disasters, flooding, and water damage: Mold and dampness. Environmental Health and Preventive Medicine. 2014;**19**(2):93-99

[46] Kanchongkittiphon W, Mendell MJ, Gaffin JM, Wang G, Phipatanakul W. Indoor environmental exposures and exacerbation of asthma: An update to the 2000 review by the Institute of Medicine. Environmental Health Perspectives. 2015;**123**(1):6-20

[47] Tischer C, Chen CM, Heinrich J. Association between domestic mould and mould components, and asthma and allergy in children: A systematic review. The European Respiratory Journal. 2011;**38**(4):812-824

[48] Jaakkola JJK, Hwang B-F, Jaakkola N. Home dampness and molds, parental atopy, and asthma in childhood: A six-year population-based cohort study. Environmental Health Perspectives. 2004;**113.3**:357-361

[49] Tischer C et al. Predictors of microbial agents in dust and respiratory health in the Ecrhs. BMC Pulmonary Medicine. 2015;**15**(1):48

[50] Biagini JM et al. Environmental risk factors of rhinitis in early infancy. Pediatric Allergy and Immunology. 2006;**17**(4):278-284

[51] Iossifova YY et al. Mold exposure during infancy as a predictor of potential asthma development. Annals of Allergy, Asthma & Immunology. 2009;**102**(2):131-137

[52] Iossifova YY et al. House dust (1-3)-β-d-glucan and wheezing in infants. Allergy. 2007;**62**(5):504-513

[53] Reponen T et al. Infant origins of childhood asthma associated with specific molds. The Journal of Allergy and Clinical Immunology. 2012;**130**(3):639-644.e5

[54] Eduard W. The Nordic Expert Group for Criteria Documentation of Health Risks from Chemicals: 139. Fungal Spores. Arbete Och Halsa; 2006;**21**:1-145

[55] Adan OCG. On the Fungal Defacement of Interior Finishes. Eindhoven University of Technology; 1994

[56] Foarde KK, Van Osdell DW, Chang JCS. Evaluation of fungal growth on fiberglass duct materials for various moisture, soil, use, and temperature conditions. Indoor Air. 1996;**6**(2):83-92

[57] Viitanen H, Ojanen T. Improved model to predict mold growth in building materials. In: ASHRAE/Proc., 10th Int. Conf. on Thermal Performance of the Exterior Envelopes of Whole Buildings X. Clearwater Beach, USA; 2-7 December 2007

[58] Hoang CP, Kinney KA, Corsi RL, Szaniszlo PJ. Resistance of green building materials to fungal growth. International Biodeterioration and Biodegradation. 2010;**64**(2):104-113

[59] Nielsen KF, Holm G, Uttrup LP, Nielsen PA. Mould growth on building materials under low water activities. Influence of humidity and temperature on fungal growth and secondary metabolism. International Biodeterioration and Biodegradation. 2004;**54**(4):325-336

[60] Klamer M, Morsinga E, Husemoenb T. Fungal growth on different insulation materials exposed to different moisture regimes. International Biodeterioration and Biodegradation. 2004;**54**(4):277-282

[61] Górny RL et al. Fungal fragments as indoor air biocontaminants. Applied and Environmental Microbiology. 2002;**68**(7):3522-3531

[62] Górny RL, Reponen T, Willeke K, Robine E, Boissier M, Grinshpun SA. Release of fungal fragments from moldy surfaces. Applied and Environmental Microbiology. 2002;**68**:3522-3531

[63] Madsen AM, Kruse P, Schneider T. Characterization of microbial particle release from biomass and building material surfaces for inhalation exposure risk assessment. The Annals of Occupational Hygiene. 2006;**50**(2):175-187

[64] Morse R, Acker D. Indoor air quality and mold prevention of the building envelope. National Institute of Building Sciences. 2009;**1**:2009

[65] Odom JD, DuBose G. Commissioning Buildings in Hot, Humid Climates: Design and Construction Guidelines. West Palm Beach, FL: Morse Zehnter Associates, The Fairmont Press, Inc.; 2000

[66] Warscheid T. Mold remediation in West-European buildings. Fundamentals of Mold Growth in Indoor Environments and Strategies for Healthy Living. Wageningen, Utrecht, The Netherlands: Wageningen Academic Publishers; 2011. pp. 413-433

[67] Kemp PC, Neumeister-Kemp HG, Esposito B, Lysek G, Murray F. Changes in airborne fungi from the outdoors

to indoor air; large HVAC systems in nonproblem buildings in two different climates. AIHA Journal. 2003;**64**(2):269-275

[68] Adan OCG. The Fungal Resistance of Interior Finishing Materials. Wageningen, Utrecht, The Netherlands: Wageningen Academic Publishers; 2011. pp. 335-352

[69] Rowan NJ, Johnstone CM, McLean RC, Anderson JG, Clarke JA. Prediction of toxigenic fungal growth in buildings by using a novel modelling system. Applied and Environmental Microbiology. 1999;**65**(11):4814-4821

[70] Grant C, Hunter CA, Flannigan B, Bravery AF. The moisture requirements of moulds isolated from domestic dwellings. International Biodeterioration. 1989;**25**(4):259-284

[71] Pasanen AL, Rautiala S, Kasanen JE, Raunio P, Rantamaki J, Kalliokosk P. The relationship between measured moisture conditions and fungal concentrations in water-damaged building materials. Indoor Air. 2000;**10**(2):111-120

[72] Dillon HK, Heinsohn PA, Miller JD. Field Guide for the Determination of Biological Contaminants in Environmental Samples. Fairfax, VA, USA: AIHA; 2005

[73] Miller JD. Mycological investigations of indoor environments. In: Microorganisms in Home and Indoor Work Environments: Diversity, Health Impacts, Investigation and Control. Vol. 2. 2011

[74] D'Souza TM, Merritt CS, Reddy CA. Lignin-modifying enzymes of the white rot basidiomycete Ganoderma lucidum. Applied and Environmental Microbiology. 1999;**65**(12):5307-5313

[75] Sedlbauer K. Prediction of mould fungus formation on the surface of and inside building components. [Thesis]. Stuttgart: Fraunhofer Institute for Building Physics; 2001

[76] Zak JC, Wildman HG. Fungi in stressful environments. In: Biodiversity of Fungi. Inventory and Monitoring Methods. London: Elsevier/Academic; 2004. pp. 303-315

[77] Kubicek CP, Esser K, Druzhinina IS. Environmental and Microbial Relationships. Vol. 4. Heidelberg, Germany: Springer Science & Business Media; 2007

[78] Nofal M, Kumaran MK. Durability assessments of wood-frame construction using the concept of damage-functions. In: Lacasse M, Vainer D, editors. Proceedings of the 8th International Conference Durability of Building Materials and Components. Vancouver, Canada; 1999. pp. 766-799

[79] Shelton BG, Kirkland KH, Flanders WD, Morris GK. Profiles of airborne fungi in buildings and outdoor environments in the United States. Applied and Environmental Microbiology. 2002;**68**(4):1743-1753

[80] Rantamaki J et al. Mould in Buildings and Building Materials. Finnish. Vol. 2000. Espoo, Finland: VTT Tied; 2000. p. 40

[81] Viitanen H et al. Moisture and bio-deterioration risk of building materials and structures. Journal of Building Physics. 2010;**33**(3):201-224

[82] Anagnost SE. Wood in the built environment: Conditions for mold and decay. In: Yang CS, Heinsohn PA, editors. Sampling and Analysis of Indoor Microorganisms. New York: John Wiley & Sons; 2007. pp. 155-178

[83] Pasanen A-L et al. Fungal growth and survival in building materials under fluctuating moisture and temperature conditions. International Biodeterioration and Biodegradation. 2000;**46**(2):117-127

[84] Andersen B, Frisvad JC, Søndergaard I, Rasmussen IS, Larsen LS. Associations between fungal species and water-damaged building materials. Applied and Environmental Microbiology. 2011;**77**(12):4180-4188

[85] Hyvärinen A, Meklin T, Vepsäläinena A, Nevalainena A. Fungi and actinobacteria in moisture-damaged building materials - concentrations and diversity. International Biodeterioration and Biodegradation. 2002;**49**(1):27-37

[86] Hukka A. A mathematical model of mould growth on wooden material. Wood Science and Technology. 2000;**33**:475-485

[87] Viitanen HA. Factors Affecting Mould Growth on Kiln Dried Wood. In: 3rd Workshop on Softwood Drying to Specific End Uses, Cost Action E 15, Advances in the Drying of Wood. Helsinki: VTT, Otawood; Vol. 4, 11-13 June 2001. pp. 1-8

[88] Meklin T et al. Quantitative PCR analysis of house dust can reveal abnormal mold conditions. Journal of Environmental Monitoring. 2004;**6**(7):615-620

[89] Crawford JA, Rosenbaum PF, Anagnost SE, Hunt A, Abraham JL. Indicators of airborne fungal concentrations in urban homes: Understanding the conditions that affect indoor fungal exposures. Science of the Total Environment. 2015;**517**:113-124

[90] Payne C, Woodward S, Petty JA. The softwood staining fungus Ophiostoma piceae: Influence of relative humidity, temperature and timber drying method on mycelial growth and coremiophore production in vitro and on wood. Journal of the Institute of Wood Science. 2000;**15**(4):165-172

[91] Murtoniemi T, Nevalainen A, Hirvonen M-R. Effect of plasterboard composition on stachybotrys chartarum growth and biological activity of spores. Applied and Environmental Microbiology. 2003;**69**(7):3751-3757

[92] Mueller A et al. Individual and combined effects of mycotoxins from typical indoor moulds. Toxicology in Vitro. 2013;**27**(6):1970-1978

[93] Webb JS, Nixon M, Eastwood IM, Greenhalgh M, Robson GD, Handley PS. Fungal colonization and biodeterioration of plasticized polyvinyl chloride. Applied and Environmental Microbiology. 2000;**66**(8):3194-3200

[94] Chang JCS. Growth evaluation of Fungi (Penicillium and Aspergillus spp.) on ceiling tiles. Atmospheric Environment. 1995;**29**(17):2331

[95] Rintala H, Pitkaranta M, Taubel M. Microbial communities associated with house dust. Advances in Applied Microbiology. 2012;**78**:75-120

[96] Kowalski WJ, Bahnfleth WP, Whittam TS. Filtration of airborne microorganisms: Modeling and prediction. ASHRAE Transactions. 1999;**105**:4-17

[97] Bridge P, Spooner B. Soil fungi: Diversity and detection. Plant and Soil. 2001;**232**(1-2):147-154

[98] Corsi RL, Siegel JA, Chiang C. Particle resuspension during the use of vacuum cleaners on residential carpet. Journal of Occupational and Environmental Hygiene. 2008;**5**(4):232-238

[99] Gomes C, Freihaut J, Bahnfleth W. Resuspension of allergen-containing particles under mechanical and aerodynamic disturbances from human walking.

Atmospheric Environment. 2007;**41**(25):5257-5270

[100] Knibbs LD, He C, Duchaine C, Morawska L. Vacuum cleaner emissions as a source of indoor exposure to airborne particles and bacteria. Environmental Science & Technology. 2011;**46**(1):534-542

[101] Qian J, Peccia J, Ferro AR. Walking-induced particle resuspension in indoor environments. Atmospheric Environment. 2014;**89**:464-481

[102] Rosati JA, Thornburg J, Rodes C. Resuspension of particulate matter from carpet due to human activity. Aerosol Science and Technology. 2008;**42**(6):472-482

[103] Veillette M et al. Microbial contents of vacuum cleaner bag dust and emitted bioaerosols and their implications for human exposure indoors. Applied and Environmental Microbiology. 2013;**79**(20): 6331-6336

[104] Afanou KA et al. Submicronic fungal bioaerosols: High-resolution microscopic characterization and quantification. Applied and Environmental Microbiology. 2014;**80**(22):7122-7130

[105] Afanou, Komlavi Anani, et al. Profile and morphology of fungal aerosols characterized by field emission scanning electron microscopy (FESEM). Aerosol Science and Technology. 2015;**496**:423-435

[106] Madsen AM, Wilkins CK, Poulsen OM. Micro-particles from fungi. In: Bioaerosols Fungi Bact. Mycotoxins Hum. Heal. Pathophysiol. Clin. Eff. Expo. Assess. Prev. Control Indoor Environ. NY: Boyd Print. Co.; 2005. pp. 276-291

[107] Reponen T, Seo S-C, Grimsley F, Lee T, Crawford C, Grinshpun SA. Fungal fragments in moldy houses: A field study in homes in New Orleans and Southern Ohio. Atmospheric Environment. 2007;**41**(37):8140-8149

[108] Foto M, Vrijmoed LLP, Miller JD, Ruest K, Lawton M, Dales RE. A comparison of airborne ergosterol, glucan and Air-O-Cell data in relation to physical assessments of mold damage and some other parameters. Indoor Air. 2005;**15**(4):257-266

[109] Green BJ, Schmechel D, Tovey ER. Detection of aerosolized Alternaria alternata conidia, hyphae, and fragments by using a novel double-immunostaining technique. Clinical and Diagnostic Laboratory Immunology. 2005;**12**(9):1114-1116

[110] Kildesø J et al. Determination of fungal spore release from wet building materials. Indoor Air. 2003;**13**(2):148-155

[111] Li D-W, Kendrick B. A year-round comparison of fungal spores in indoor and outdoor air. Mycologia. 1995;**87**:190-195

[112] Adhikari A, Reponen T, Rylander R. Airborne fungal cell fragments in homes in relation to total fungal biomass. Indoor Air. 2013;**23**(2):142-147

[113] Kanaani H, Hargreaves M, Smith J, Ristovski Z, Agranovski V, Morawska L. Performance of UVAPS with respect to detection of airborne fungi. Journal of Aerosol Science. 2008;**39**(2):175-189

[114] Miller JD, Rand TG, Jarvis BB. Stachybotrys chartarum: Cause of human disease or media darling? Medical Mycology. 2003;**41**(4):271-291

[115] Green BJ et al. Surveillance of fungal allergic sensitization using the fluorescent halogen immunoassay.

Journal De Mycologie Medicale/ Journal of Medical Mycology. 2009;**19**(4):253-261

[116] Green BJ, Sercombe JK, Tovey ER. Fungal fragments and undocumented conidia function as new aeroallergen sources. The Journal of Allergy and Clinical Immunology. 2005;**115**(5):1043-1048

[117] Brasel TL, Douglas DR, Wilson SC, Straus DC. Detection of airborne Stachybotrys chartarum macrocyclic trichothecene mycotoxins on particulates smaller than conidia. Applied and Environmental Microbiology. 2005;**71**(1):114-122

[118] Penttinen P, Timonen KL, Tiittanen P, Mirme A, Ruuskanen J, Pekkanen J. Ultrafine particles in urban air and respiratory health among adult asthmatics. The European Respiratory Journal. 2001;**17**(3):428-435

[119] von Klot S et al. Increased asthma medication use in association with ambient fine and ultrafine particles. The European Respiratory Journal. 2002;**20**(3):691-702

[120] Saari S et al. Effects of fungal species, cultivation time, growth substrate, and air exposure velocity on the fluorescence properties of airborne fungal spores. Indoor Air. 2015;**25**(6):653-661

[121] Mensah-Attipoe J et al. Release and characteristics of fungal fragments in various conditions. Science of the Total Environment. 2016;**547**:234-243

[122] Agranovski V, Ristovski Z, Blackall PJ, Morawska L. Size-selective assessment of airborne particles in swine confinement building with the UVAPS. Atmospheric Environment. 2004;**38**(23):3893-3901

[123] Healy DA, Huffman JA, O'Connor DJ, Pöhlker C, Pöschl U, Sodeau JR. Ambient measurements of biological aerosol particles near Killarney, Ireland: A comparison between real-time fluorescence and microscopy techniques. Atmospheric Chemistry and Physics. 2014;**14**(15):8055-8069

[124] Seo S-C, Reponen T, Levin L, Grinshpun SA. Size-fractionated (1 → 3)-β-D-glucan concentrations aerosolized from different moldy building materials. Science of the Total Environment. 2009;**407**(2):806-814

[125] Kanaani H, Hargreaves M, Ristovski Z, Morawska L. Performance assessment of UVAPS: Influence of fungal spore age and air exposure. Journal of Aerosol Science. 2007;**38**(1):83-96

Chapter 5

High Incidence of an Emerging Opportunistic Pathogen *Candida parapsilosis* in Water-Related Domestic Environments

Jerneja Zupančič, Monika Novak Babič and Nina Gunde-Cimerman

Abstract

Candidiasis is one of the common fungal opportunistic infections, usually associated with diverse *Candida* species. *Candida albicans*, *C. glabrata* complex, *C. parapsilosis* complex, *C. tropicalis* and *C. auris* are often identified in affected patients. *Candida parapsilosis* sensu stricto is an emerging cause of hospital-acquired Candida infections, predominantly in Southern Europe, South America and Asia. Home environment is a less known source of infection despite frequent isolation of *C. parapsilosis* from kitchen surfaces and household appliances such as dishwashers, washing machines and refrigerators. *C. parapsilosis* is one of the first colonisers of novel dishwashers and a member of stable fungal communities on rubber seals worldwide in concentrations up to 10^2 CFU/cm^2. It colonises also drawers for detergents in washing machines and drainage channels in refrigerators. Tap water and groundwater act as vector for entrance of *C. parapsilosis* in the indoor environments. Within *C. parapsilosis*, four clinically relevant phenotypes can be distinguished. Experimental data on the prevalence of *C. parapsilosis* isolates phenotypes, obtained from indoor environments, will be presented. Smooth phenotype prevails in dishwashers and washing machines, while crepe and crater dominate in water. In conclusion, the ability to colonise diverse environments and accordingly switch phenotypes defines *C. parapsilosis* as a versatile, domestic environment-related opportunistic pathogen.

Keywords: emerging opportunistic pathogen, water, household appliances, phenotype occurrence in domestic environments

1. Introduction

Yeast *Candida parapsilosis* sensu stricto (Ascomycota, Saccharomycetes, Saccharomycetales, Debaryomycetaceae) is the most commonly isolated species from *C. parapsilosis* complex, followed by its closest relative *C. orthopsilosis* and *C. metapsilosis* [1]. Its primary natural habitat remains undefined to date although it was recently reported from different fresh water sources [2–4] as well as from pine trees [5]. On the other hand, the presence of *C. parapsilosis* in relation to humans is well documented [1, 6]. The species is one of the asymptomatic colonisers of gastrointestinal and reproductive tract of most healthy humans [6]. In addition, it is commonly found on the skin and nails [1, 6]. Thus, the carriage and transfer of *C. parapsilosis* via hands of healthcare workers to patients have been for long recognised as a cause of opportunistic infections in hospitals [7]. The significance and prevalence of the yeast in clinical settings and samples dramatically increased during the past two decades, which ranks it among emerging opportunistic human pathogens [8]. *C. parapsilosis* is globally one of the most frequent non-albicans *Candida* (NAC) species causing a broad spectrum of infections from superficial to invasive candidiasis, including vulvovaginal infections, nosocomial bloodstream infections, pericarditis, endocarditis, endophthalmitis and sepsis [1, 9–12]. Individuals at the highest risk for severe infection include neonates and patients in intensive care units [8]. Infections with *C. parapsilosis* are often related to contaminated catheters, due to its remarkable ability to produce biofilms on plastic and silicone surfaces of catheter instruments [6, 8, 13]. Ability for successful biofilm formation was linked with observed phenotypic differences of *C. parapsilosis* strains [14]. Among four described phenotypes (smooth, crepe, crater and concentric), the yeastlike smooth phenotype reportedly formed less biofilm in comparison to the entirely filamentous concentric phenotype [14].

In our study we focused on little known phenotypic diversity of *C. parapsilosis* strains, isolated from clinical material in comparison to those isolated from human-made indoor environments, particularly related to tap water and household appliances, such as washing machines, dishwashers and refrigerators. In addition, we discuss the ability for biofilm formation among tested strains and possible sources of infection originating from the household environment.

2. Daily home-related activities pose an overlooked infection risk

The risk for infection caused by *C. parapsilosis* is reportedly the highest in hospitals and healthcare facilities, as *C. parapsilosis* is commonly transferred via hands of healthcare workers [1, 7]. However, recent discoveries reveal domestic environments as sites where people are exposed to this emerging pathogen on a daily basis. Exposure points include water and hygiene-related activities, cooking area and household appliances, like dishwashers, washing machines and refrigerators. *C. parapsilosis* was isolated in high frequencies from these areas, pointing towards its preference for indoor environment [4, 15–18].

2.1 Water as a vector for transmission of *Candida parapsilosis* into household environment

In a modern society, microbiologically safe and potable water is not only one of the essential human rights but also remains one of the biggest concerns for the future [19]. Despite well-established water cleaning procedures, both, filamentous fungi and yeasts, are widely present in water intended for human consumption [19]. Except Swedish legislation, fungal parameters are not included in the present directives, and the lack of monitoring leaves out opportunistic and emerging fungal pathogens [19]. During the last 10 years, different water sources were identified as vectors for *C. parapsilosis*. Raw natural water, contaminated with *C. parapsilosis*, included streams [2], rivers [3], and groundwater [4]. Its presence positively correlated with the occurrence of dry season [3], the presence of middle-hard water type and nitrates [4, 18, 20]. Due to its ability to withstand filtration and chlorination process [21], *C. parapsilosis* is one of the building blocks in biofilms within municipal water systems, with the number of yeast cells in a range of 3.1–4.6 CFU/cm^2 [22].

Consequently, *C. parapsilosis* is regularly present in tap water at consumers' points, where it was isolated from 11 to 50% of samples [4, 17, 21, 23, 24]. Taps need thus to be taken into consideration as one of the important exposure points in households, where people may become infected with *C. parapsilosis* via drinking, food preparation and personal hygiene, like showering and bathing [19, 25].

2.2 Kitchens without dishwashers more likely host *Candida parapsilosis*

In every household, preparation and consumption of food cause dirty dishes, which can be cleaned manually or in a dishwasher. During the cleaning of kitchen utensils, the prewashing and washing steps are usually carried out using sponges in order to remove food residues. In due course, some food residues could adhere to the sponges and, together with retained humidity, tender a positive environment for growth and survival of pathogenic bacteria [26] and yeasts [27], including *C. parapsilosis*. From a microbiological point of view, kitchen surfaces are one of the most contaminated environments of our homes [17, 28–30]. Kitchen surfaces are not aseptic, but with proper cleaning, microorganisms may be reduced to the level that is generally recognised as safe. The most probable entryways of *C. parapsilosis* into domestic kitchen are water [4, 17] and human skin [15]. Adams et al. [15] reported that the highest incidence of C. parapsilosis is on the skin of the inhabitants (40%) and kitchen drains (25%) but the same yeast has a very low settle index on windowsills in kitchens (up to 2%). Zupančič et al. [17] reported the presence of *C. parapsilosis* on kitchen surfaces in high frequencies (up to 77% of tested kitchen surfaces were populated with *C. parapsilosis*). However, fungal diversity and occurrence varied considerably between kitchens containing dishwasher and kitchens without. The most significant difference was the presence of *C. parapsilosis*, which strongly dominated kitchens using handwashing only. The most contaminated sites in these kitchens were drain (43%), followed by dish drying rack and sink in the same occurrence (36%). Settlement index of *C. parapsilosis* on rubber seal in kitchen drain and kitchen counter did not exceed 25% [17].

2.3 *Candida parapsilosis* is the first coloniser of new dishwashers

In modern societies, dishwashers are a permanent utility in kitchens facilitating residents' daily tasks. Washing in a dishwasher is usually carried out at high temperatures of 55–65°C, followed by a shorter hot water rinse cycle (~85°C) and the use of alkaline detergents. The mechanical power of water jets cleans the vessels [31]. The dishwashers do not disinfect the dishes, but reduce the number of microorganisms to a level that is considered safe [32]. The number of bacteria on the vessels is partly reduced due to high pH and temperature [33]. Recent studies have shown that under these unfavourable conditions, such as high temperature, wet and dry periods, high and low pH, presence of high concentrations of salt (NaCl) and water shearing forces, a certain group of microorganisms—polyextremotolerant ones—are enriched [34]. These unfavourable circumstances can defy also the opportunistic pathogenic species like *C. parapsilosis* [17], which seems to be one of the first colonisers of new dishwashers [20], providing a biotic surface for the construction of mixed bacterial-fungal biofilms [35]. *C. parapsilosis* forms together with *Exophiala dermatitidis*, *Exophiala phaeomuriformis*, *Rhodotorula mucilaginosa*, *Aureobasidium melanogenum*, *Bisifusarium dimerum* (formerly *Fusarium dimerum*), *Fusarium oxysporum* and *Saprochaete clavata*, a stable microbiota of dishwasher rubber seals worldwide [17, 34, 36, 37]. It is globally present on rubber seals of dishwashers [34, 36] with settlement up to 10^2 CFU/cm^2 [17]. It can be found in high frequencies also on dishwasher doors and walls. Drains, cutlery racks and side nozzles are less exposed [17]. Higher dishwasher frequency of use (7–14 times per week) and connection to tap water system with moderately hard tap water hardness (1.5–2 mmol/l $CaCO_3$) significantly affect the incidence of *C. parapsilosis* [20]. *C. parapsilosis* can be released from dishwashers via waste water, cleaned vessels and hot aerosols, formed at the end of the washing cycle [17].

2.4 The use of softeners increases the likelihood of *Candida parapsilosis* settlement inside washing machines

Knowledge on washing machines' microbiomes is relevant particularly in hospitals and other healthcare facilities due to the possible transfer of pathogenic microorganisms between clothes being washed at the same time [38, 39]. Washing cycles at elevated temperatures may prevent cross-contamination lowering the number of microorganisms, but recent energy-saving trends promote washing with biodegradable detergents and usage of eco-programmes with temperatures of washing not exceeding 40°C [16]. These features favour microbial growth and propagation, resulting in persistent odour of textiles and elevated risk for infections [39, 40]. The main worries remain the bacteria of the genera *Pseudomonas* and *Staphylococcus*, together with dermatophyte fungi [38]. However, recent studies conducted globally reported *C. parapsilosis* as one of the most common fungi in washing machines, colonising 8–25% of sampled machines [16, 18, 41]. It was isolated mainly from biofilms at water-entry points, drawers for detergent and softener and rubber seals [16, 18, 41]. Its presence in washing machines positively correlated with the regular use of commercial softeners and washing temperatures ≤40°C [16]. Forty-eight percent of tested *C. parapsilosis* strains from washing machines showed a remarkable ability of biofilm formation, while none of the tested strains grew on 0.1% cycloheximide [18].

2.5 *Candida parapsilosis* colonises refrigerators' rubber and moist parts

Primarily basidiomycetous yeasts but to a lesser extent also ascomycetous yeasts have been reported from extremely cold natural environments, including *C. parapsilosis* [42]. Extremely cold environments are also present indoors, in the form of refrigerators and freezers. Until date, there are no reports of yeasts, isolated from freezers, and few are reporting their isolation from refrigerators. Yeasts have been isolated from plastic refrigerator vegetable compartments, rubber seals, walls and water dispensers [43, 44]. *Candida* species have been isolated most frequently, with *Pichia kudriavzevii* prevailing in refrigerator air [45]. Our preliminary results showed the presence of *C. parapsilosis* on the shelves and in drainage channel of domestic refrigerators.

3. Phenotypic diversity of *Candida parapsilosis* in domestic environments

Phenotypic diversity of *C. parapsilosis* was first described by Enger et al. [46] who identified five different phenotypes originating from one isolate (crepe, concentric, snowball, rough and smooth) [46]. They were later reidentified into four groups, crepe, concentric, smooth and crater, with a described ability to switch from one phenotype into another [14]. Phenotypic differences of the strains were linked with micromorphological features, growth rate and the ability to form biofilm [14]. The yeast cells of smooth phenotype grow most rapidly but form less biofilm in comparison to the crepe or crater phenotype. On the other hand, concentric phenotype produces entirely filamentous cells and forms biofilm most successfully (**Table 1**) [14].

Phenotype properties	Phenotypes			
	Crepe	Crater	Concentric	Smooth
Micromorphology	Pseudohyphae	Elongated, yeastlike	Wide, pseudohyphae	Small, yeastlike
Chitin distribution	Cell wall	Cell wall, bud neck	Cell wall, bud neck	Bud scar
Growth rate	Medium	Medium	Low	High
Biofilm formation ability	Medium	Medium	High	Low

Table 1.
The main differences between four phenotypic groups of ***C. parapsilosis*** *according to Laffey and Butler (2005) [14].*

3.1 Smooth phenotype of *Candida parapsilosis* prevails in domestic environment

One-hundred and eighty-four strains of *C. parapsilosis* sensu lato, deposited in Ex Culture Collection of the Infrastructural Centre Mycosmo, MRIC UL, Slovenia: http://www.ex-genebank.com/, at the Department of Biology, Biotechnical Faculty, University of Ljubljana, were included in the present study. Tested strains originated from clinical material (N = 7), groundwater (N = 2) and domestic environment, like tap water (N = 23), bathrooms (N = 14), washing machines (N = 16), kitchens (N = 22), dishwashers (N = 96) and refrigerators (N = 4). All strains were plated onto malt extract agar and incubated at 30°C for 4 weeks. Phenotypic diversity of the strains (**Figure 1**) was evaluated weekly (**Table 2**).

Identification of yeasts from the *C. parapsilosis* complex can often be false or incorrect, since the species *C. parapsilosis*, *C. metapsilosis* and *C. orthopsilosis* are genetically very similar. Commercially available reagents currently do not allow accurate distinction within the *C. parapsilosis* complex [47]. One of the methods

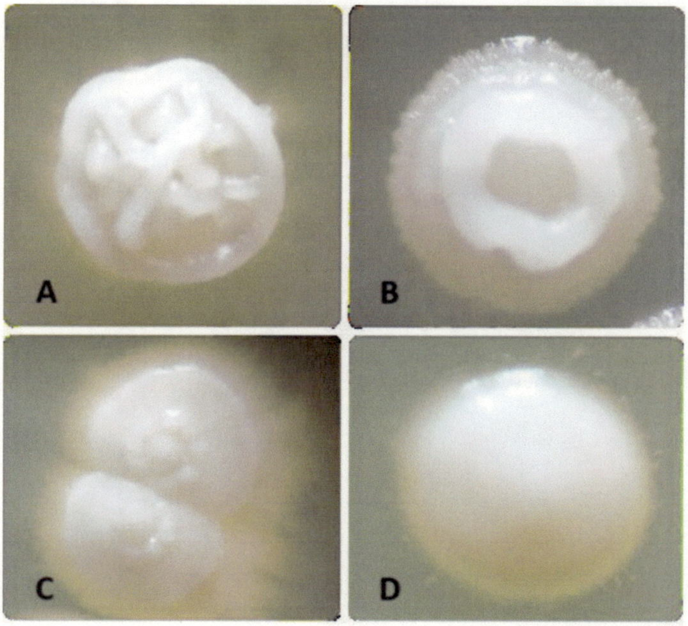

Figure 1.
C. parapsilosis phenotypes in domestic environment. (A) Crepe phenotype, (B) concentric phenotype, (C) crater phenotype and (D) smooth phenotype.

		Environment							
		Clinical material	Groundwater	Tap water	Bathroom	Washing machine	Kitchen	Dishwasher	Refrigerator
Phenotypes	Crepe	EXF-10095; EXF-10098; EXF-10192; EXF-10193;	EXF-8460; EXF-8247	EXF-8404; EXF-8405; EXF-8452; EXF-9873; EXF-10048	EXF-12615; EXF-12765	EXF-6337; EXF-8239	EXF-9920 EXF-9924 EXF-9925 EXF-9954 EXF-9574	EXF-8850; EXF-8854; EXF-8862; EXF-8907; EXF-8908; EXF-8909; EXF-8931; EXF-9096; EXF-9103; EXF-9105; EXF-9108; EXF-9112; EXF-9113; EXF-9190; EXF-9193; EXF-9207; EXF-9220; EXF-9251; EXF-9259; EXF-9311; EXF-9354; EXF-9355; EXF-9384; EXF-9386; EXF-9490; EXF-9491	EXF-9596
	Crater	EXF-10096		EXF-9872; EXF-10133; EXF-10144; EXF-10179; EXF-10240; EXF-9623; EXF-9693	EXF-12671; EXF-9692		EXF-9915 EXF-9960 EXF-12806	EXF-8892; EXF-8901; EXF-8905; EXF-8914; EXF-9081; EXF-9092; EXF-9106; EXF-9110; EXF-9330; EXF-9334	
	Concentric	EXF-10099		EXF-5670; EXF-8411; EXF-8248	EXF-6998	EXF-6334	EXF-9941; EXF-9952; EXF-9953; EXF-10087; EXF-8104	EXF-6078; EXF-8903; EXF-8937; EXF-8938; EXF-9045; EXF-9048; EXF-9099; EXF-9260; EXF-9280; EXF-9281; EXF-9283; EXF-9326; EXF-9342; EXF-9361; EXF-9389; EXF-9475; EXF-9496	

	Environment							
	Clinical material	**Groundwater**	**Tap water**	**Bathroom**	**Washing machine**	**Kitchen**	**Dishwasher**	**Refrigerator**
Smooth	EXF-10097		EXF-8406; EXF-9899; EXF-10058; EXF-10067; EXF-10174; EXF-9691; EXF-9694; EXF-9697	EXF-6342; EXF-6356; EXF-7001; EXF-12776; EXF-9696; EXF-8101; EXF-8146; EXF-8149	EXF-5667; EXF-5730; EXF-5731; EXF-8288; EXF-8289; EXF-8290; EXF-8296; EXF-9781; EXF-9782; EXF-6335; EXF-6336; EXF-6338; EXF-8399	EXF-9907; EXF-9916; EXF-9928; EXF-9944; EXF-9955; EXF-9956 EXF-8111; EXF-9556 EXF-9557	EXF-8251; EXF-5540; EXF-5545; EXF-5547; EXF-5659; EXF-5717; EXF-5722; EXF-5723; EXF-5726; EXF-5728; EXF-6088; EXF-6102; EXF-6112; EXF-6120; EXF-6126; EXF-8849; EXF-8866; EXF-8867; EXF-8894; EXF-8919; EXF-9052; EXF-9054; EXF-9088; EXF-9095; EXF-9102; EXF-9200; EXF-9203; EXF-9206; EXF-9224; EXF-9275; EXF-9278; EXF-9340; EXF-9364; EXF-9370; EXF-9371; EXF-9395; EXF-9504; EXF-9509; EXF-9514; EXF-9535; EXF-9537; EXF-9769; EXF-9211	EXF-11755; EXF-12203; EXF-12266

Table 2.
Phenotypic diversity of ***C. parapsilosis*** *sensu stricto strains. EXF refers to culture collection strain designation.*

used for genetic differentiation between the complex species is also the analysis of the restriction polymorphism of the secondary alcohol dehydrogenase (*SADH*) gene [48]. After DNA extraction, identification based on the whole internal transcribed spacer (ITS) region and partial 28S rDNA, D1/D2 domains, was performed. All tested strains were checked for accurate identification of *C. parapsilosis* species complex by RFLP analyses of the *SADH* gene fragment. *SADH* amplicons obtained with the primer set S1F and S1R [49] were digested with the restriction enzyme *Ban*I. All tested strains belonged to *C. parapsilosis* sensu stricto group.

Obtained results showed differences between abundance of phenotypes in clinical strains in comparison to the environmental strains (**Figure 2**). The prevalent phenotype among clinical strains was crepe (57.1%), while the others were evenly distributed (14.3%). The results are similar to already reported by Laffey and Butler [14]. Among environmental strains, the crepe phenotype was the only one observed in strains isolated from groundwater (2/2). It was represented in a lesser extent in household appliances, with the highest incidence on kitchen surfaces (22.7%) and in dishwashers (27.1%), and the lowest in washing machines (12.5%).

C. parapsilosis strains isolated from groundwater-derived tap water mostly formed smooth (34.8%) or crater (30.4%) phenotypes, followed by crepe (21.7%) and concentric (13.0%) phenotype. Tap water serves as a vector for fungi entering water-related niches in households [4], where environmental pressure leads to the selection of the most tolerant strains [17], even on the phenotypic level. Room interior and household appliances that are usually present in these rooms (bathroom and washing machine, kitchen and dishwasher) show similar phenotype distribution (**Figure 3**). In addition, co-occurrence of different phenotypes from

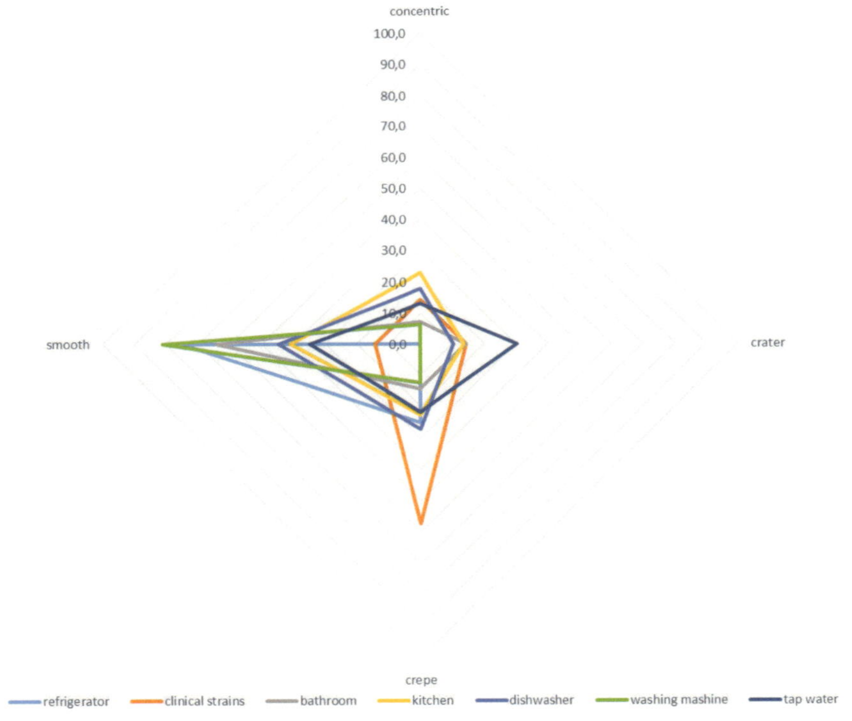

Figure 2.
Prevalence of C. parapsilosis phenotype in indoor environments and among clinical isolates. Prevailing indoor phenotype of C. parapsilosis is the smooth one; crepe phenotype is a predominant phenotype in clinical isolates.

DOI: http://dx.doi.org/10.5772/intechopen.81313

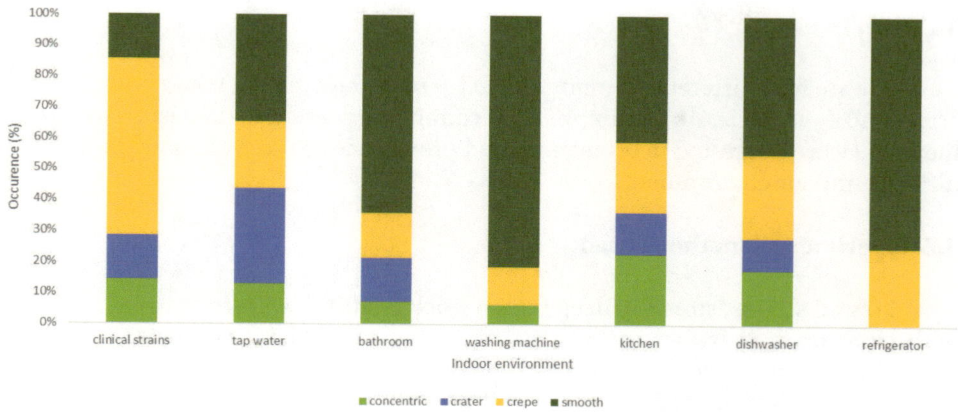

Figure 3.
Distribution of C. parapsilosis phenotypes in indoor environments. In clinical strains, crepe phenotype was prevailing, while in household appliances, such as washing machines, dishwashers and refrigerators, the predominant phenotype was smooth. Crepe phenotype was present to a lesser extent.

the same sampling spot was observed. Smooth phenotype was positively selected in all appliances, washing machine, refrigerator and dishwasher, with 81.3, 75.0 and 44.8%, respectively. Slightly positive selection was observed also for concentric phenotype in kitchens (22.7%) and inside dishwashers (17.7%) in comparison to bathrooms (7.1%) and washing machines (6.3%). On the other hand, negative selection was observed for crater phenotype, which was among all tested habitats most commonly found in tap water (30.4%), but its presence was low on kitchen (13.6%) and bathroom (14.3%) surfaces, with total absence in washing machines and refrigerators.

Survival of microorganisms invading household niches is higher due to biofilm formation [17]. Next-generation sequencing of dishwasher biofilm community and further usage of several statistical models showed that *Candida* (*C. parapsilosis*) is one of the first colonisers of rubber seals in dishwashers [20].

4. Conclusions

C. parapsilosis is a commonly known opportunistic pathogen, particularly in a connection with hospital care, as a natural coloniser of health workers' hands and skin. Superficial or invasive infections usually occur via catheters, due to yeast's biofilm formation ability. Recent studies revealed human-made indoor environments as a previously unrecognised hot spot of their occurrence. This completely new aspect enables many possible routes for infection with this emerging opportunistic pathogen. *C. parapsilosis* is commonly present in tap water, bathrooms, washing machines, kitchens surfaces, dishwashers and refrigerators. While tap water carried all four phenotypes of the species, with a slight preference for the crater phenotype, selection inside household appliances clearly promoted the smooth phenotype. In accordance, the smooth phenotype showed the most abundant biofilm formation on polystyrene. On the other hand, tested clinical strains mainly formed the crepe phenotype, which was isolated also from all sampled indoor niches, with the highest incidence in kitchens, dishwashers and refrigerators. In the future, household environments where people maintain and prepare food and personal hygiene should be taken into consideration as possible routes for infection with *C. parapsilosis*.

4.1 Objectives

There are four different phenotypes of *C. parapsilosis* strains, smooth, crepe, crater and concentric. As *C. parapsilosis* is commonly present in domestic environment, we were interested in occurrence and prevalence of these phenotypes in different indoor environments.

4.2 Experimental methods used

All tested strains, stored in deep frozen stock (−80°C), were inoculated with a loop on malt extract agar plates (MEA) and incubated for 4 weeks at 30°C. Phenotype check-up was made after 1, 2, 3 and 4 weeks of incubation. Results of *C. parapsilosis* phenotype occurrence after 4 weeks are presented in **Table 2**.

4.2.1 Extraction and molecular characterisation of DNA

Pure fungal cultures were revived from deep frozen stock of EX culture collection by inoculation on a fresh malt extract agar medium. After 3 days of incubation at 30°C, the DNA was extracted using PrepMan Ultra reagent (Applied Biosystems), according to the manufacturer instructions.

Identification was based on amplification and sequencing of the large subunit ribosomal DNA sequences (LSU; partial 28S rDNA, D1/D2 domains), using the NL1 and NL4 primer set [50]. A fragment of the rDNA including internal transcribed spacer (ITS) region 1, 5.8S rDNA and ITS2 was also amplified and sequenced for identification, using the ITS5 and ITS4 primer set [51]. The ITS and LSU nucleotide sequences were determined by direct PCR sequencing, performed by Microsynth AG, Switzerland. BigDye terminator cycle sequencing kits were used in the sequence reactions (Applied Biosystems, Foster City, CA, USA). The sequences were obtained using an ABI Prism 3700 Big Dye Sequencer (Applied Biosystems). The sequences were assembled using FinchTV 1.4 (Geospiza, PerkinElmer, Inc.) and automatically and manually aligned using the Molecular Evolutionary Genetics Analysis (MEGA) software, version 6.06 [52]. The assembled DNA sequences were examined using the BLAST software of the National Center for Biotechnology Information (NCBI) database and were compared to the appropriate sequences of the reference and type strains. All strains, included into this research, were sequenced as *C. parapsilosis* sensu lato.

4.2.2 Determination of Candida parapsilosis species complex

Amplification of *SADH* gene was performed using S1F and S1R primer set according to [49]. After the final amplification, PCR products were treated with restriction enzyme *Ban*I (*BshN*I) (Thermo Fisher Scientific™, USA) according to the manufacturer instructions. After restriction the obtained fragments were checked on 1% agarose gel (Sigma-Aldrich) for 20 minutes at 120 V. The expected fragment length for *Candida metapsilosis* was 400 bp, for *Candida orthopsilosis* was 700 bp and for *Candida parapsilosis* was 550 bp [49]. After restriction profile, all tested strains were determined as *Candida parapsilosis* sensu stricto.

Acknowledgements

Infrastructural centre Mycosmo MRIC UL, the Culture Collection of Extremophilic Fungi (Ex) and Research Programme P1-0170 supported the work.

The authors would like to thank also Dr. Tadeja Matos, MD, who provided clinical strains for the study, and Daša Janeš, Mag. Biochem., for helping with the identification of the strains.

Conflict of interest

Authors declare no conflict of interest.

Author details

Jerneja Zupančič, Monika Novak Babič and Nina Gunde-Cimerman*
Department of Biology, Biotechnical Faculty, University of Ljubljana, Ljubljana, Slovenia

*Address all correspondence to: nina.gunde-cimerman@bf.uni-lj.si

References

[1] de Hoog GS, Guarro J, Gené J, Figueras MJ. Atlas of Clinical Fungi, Electronic Version 4.0. Utrecht: Centraalbureau voor Schimmelcultures; 2014. http://www.clinicalfungi.org/

[2] Ayanbimpe MG, Abbah EV, Ior AC. Yeasts and yeast-like fungal contaminants of water used for domestic purposes in Jos, Nigeria. Microbiological Research. 2012;**3**:99-102

[3] Medeiros OA, Missagia SB, Brandão RL, Callisto M, Barbosa ARF, Rosa AC. Water quality and diversity of yeasts from tropical lakes and rivers from the Rio Doce basin in Southeastern Brazil. Brazilian Journal of Microbiology. 2012;**43**(4):1582-1594

[4] Novak Babič M, Zalar P, Ženko B, Džeroski S, Gunde-Cimerman N. Yeasts and yeast-like fungi in tap water and groundwater, and their transmission to household appliances. Fungal Ecology. 2016;**20**:30-39

[5] Maganti H, Bartfai D, Xu J. Ecological structuring of yeasts associated with trees around Hamilton, Ontario, Canada. FEMS Yeast Research. 2012;**12**:9-19

[6] Suhr MJ. Characterization and investigation of fungi inhabiting the gastrointestinal tract of healthy and diseased humans [thesis]. Lincoln: University of Nebraska; 2015

[7] Huang YC, Lin TY, Leu HS, Wu JL, Chang HY. Yeast carriage on hands of hospital personnel working in intensive care units. The Journal of Hospital Infection. 1998;**39**:47-51

[8] Trofa D, Gácser A, Nosanchuk JD. *Candida parapsilosis*, an emerging fungal pathogen. Clinical Microbiology Reviews. 2008;**21**(4):606-625. DOI: 10.1128/CMR.00013-08

[9] Pfaller MA, Diekema DJ. Epidemiology of invasive candidiasis: A persistent public health problem. Clinical Microbiology Reviews. 2007;**20**(1):133-163

[10] Laal Kargar M, Fooladi-Rad S, Mohammad Davoodi M, Khalilzadeh S, Hassanzad M, Mayahi S, et al. Fungal colonization in patients with cystic fibrosis. Journal of Mazandaran University of Medical Sciences. 2013;**22**(2):204-218

[11] Bassetti M, Merelli M, Righi E, Diaz-Martin A, Rosello EM, Luzzati R, et al. Epidemiology, species distribution, antifungal susceptibility, and outcome of candidemia across five sites in Italy and Spain. Journal of Clinical Microbiology. 2013;**51**(12):4167-4172

[12] Nucci M, Queiroz-Telles F, Alvarado-Matute T, Tiraboschi IN, Cortes J, Zurita J, et al. Epidemiology of candidemia in Latin America: A laboratory-based survey. PLoS One. 2013;**8**(3):e59373. DOI: 10.1371/journal.pone.0059373

[13] Pires HR, dos Santos MJ, Zaia EJ, Gomes Martins HC, Mendes-Giannini SJM. *Candida parapsilosis* complex water isolates from a haemodialysis unit: Biofilm production and in vitro evaluation of the use of clinical antifungals. Memórias do Instituto Oswaldo Cruz. 2011;**106**(6):646-654

[14] Laffey SF, Butler G. Phenotype switching affects biofilm formation by *Candida parapsilosis*. Microbiologica. 2005;**151**:1073-1081

[15] Adams RI, Miletto M, Taylor JW, Bruns TD. The diversity and distribution of fungi on residential surfaces. PLoS One. 2013;**8**(11):e78866. DOI: 10.1371/journal.pone.0078866

[16] Novak Babič M, Zalar P, Ženko B, Schroers HJ, Džeroski S, Gunde-Cimerman N. *Candida* and *Fusarium* species known as opportunistic human pathogens from customer-accessible parts of residential washing machines. Fungal Biology. 2015;**119**:95-113. DOI: 10.1016/j.funbio.2014.10.007

[17] Zupančič J, Novak Babič M, Zalar P, Gunde-Cimerman N. The black yeast *Exophiala dermatitidis* and other selected opportunistic human fungal pathogens spread from dishwashers to kitchens. PLoS One. 2016;**11**:e014816

[18] Dögen A, Sav H, Gonca S, Kaplan E, Ilkit M, Novak Babič M, et al. *Candida parapsilosis* in domestic laundry machines. Medical Mycology. 2017;**55**(8):813-819

[19] Novak Babič M, Gunde-Cimerman N, Vargha M, Tischner Z, Magyar D, Veríssimo C, et al. Fungal contaminants in drinking water regulation? A tale of ecology, exposure, purification and clinical relevance. International Journal of Environmental Research and Public Health. 2017;**14**:636. DOI: 10.3390/ijerph14060636

[20] Raghupathi PK, Zupančič J, Brejnrod AD, Jacquiod S, Houf K, Burmølle M, Gunde-Cimerman N, Sørensen SJ. 2018. Microbial diversity and putative opportunistic pathogens in dishwasher biofilm communities. Applied and Environmental Microbiology 84:e02755-17. https://doi.org/10.1128/AEM.02755-17

[21] Shaker KB, Sharif MF. Isolation and identification of some fungi frome Al-Sader water treatment plant, Baghdad, Iraq. Al-Mustansiriyah Journal of Science. 2012;**23**(5):1-12

[22] Doggett MS. Characterisation of fungal biofilms within a municipal water distribution system. Applied and Environmental Microbiology. 2000;**66**:1249-1251. DOI: 10.1128/AEM.66.3.1249-1251.2000

[23] Yamaguchi UM, Rampazzo PCR, Yamada-Ogatta FS, Nakamura VC, Ueda-Nakamura T, del Filho DPB. Yeasts and filamentous fungi in bottled mineral water and tap water from municipal supplies. Brazilian Archives of Biology and Technology. 2007;**50**:1-9

[24] Biedunkiewicz A, Kowalska K, Schulz Ł, Stojek K, Dynowska M, Ejdys E, et al. Mycological monitoring of selected aquatic ecosystems in the context of epidemiological hazards. Drinking water. Annals of Parasitology. 2014;**60**:191-198

[25] Francesca N, Gagli R, Stucchi C, De Martino S, Moschetti G, Settanni L. Yeasts and moulds contaminants of food ice cubes and their survival in different drinks. Journal of Applied Microbiology. 2017;**124**:188-196

[26] Mattick K, Durham K, Domingue G, Jørgensen F, Sen M, Schaffner DW, et al. The survival of foodborne pathogens during domestic washing-up and subsequent transfer onto washing-up sponges, kitchen surfaces and food. International Journal of Food Microbiology. 2003;**85**(3):213-226

[27] Wolde T, Bacha K. Microbiological safety of kitchen sponges used in food establishments. International Journal of Food Sciences and Nutrition. 2016;**2016**:1659784. DOI: 10.1155/2016/1659784

[28] Ojima M, Toshima Y, Koya E, Ara K, Kawai S, Ueda N. Bacterial contamination of Japanese households and related concern about sanitation. International Journal of Environmental Health Research. 2002;**12**:41-52

[29] Sinclair RG, Gerba CP. Microbial contamination in kitchens and bathrooms of rural Cambodian

village households. Letters in Applied Microbiology. 2011;**52**:144-149

[30] Flores GE, Bates ST, Caporaso JG, Lauber CL, Leff JW, Knight R, et al. Diversity, distribution and sources of bacteria in residential kitchens. Environmental Microbiology. 2013;**15**:588-596

[31] Ståhl Wernersson E, Johansson E, Håkanson H. Cross-contamination in dishwashers. The Journal of Hospital Infection. 2004;**56**:312-317

[32] Nicolella C, Casini B, Rossi F, Chericoni A, Pardini G. Thermal sanitizing in a commercial dishwashing machine. Journal of Food Safety. 2011;**31**:81-90

[33] Jeppsson M, Ståhl Wernersson E, Håkanson H. The effect of silver ions and chlorine on the survival of *Staphylococcus aureus* and *Bacillus cereus* in dishwater. Environmental Technology. 2007;**28**:1419-1427

[34] Zalar P, Novak M, de Hoog GS, Gunde-Cimerman N. Dishwashers—A man-made ecological niche accommodating human opportunistic fungal pathogens. Fungal Biology. 2011;**115**:997-1007

[35] Zupančič J, Raghupathi PK, Houf K, Burmølle M, Sørensen SJ, Gunde-Cimerman N. Synergistic interactions in microbial biofilms facilitate the establishment of opportunistic pathogenic fungi in household dishwashers. Frontiers in Microbiology. 2018;**9**:21. DOI: 10.3389/fmicb.2018.00021

[36] Döğen A, Kaplan E, Oksüz Z, Serin MS, Ilkit M, de Hoog GS. Dishwashers are a major source of human opportunistic yeast-like fungi in indoor environments in Mersin, Turkey. Medical Mycology. 2013;**5**:493-498

[37] Gümral R, Özhak-Baysan B, Tümgör A, Saraçlı MA, Yıldıran ŞT, Ilkit M, et al. Dishwashers provide a selective extreme environment for human-opportunistic yeast-like fungi. Fungal Diversity. 2016;**76**:1-9

[38] Bloomfield SF, Exner M, Nath KJ, Scott EA, Signorelli C. The Infection Risks Associated with Clothing and Household Linens in Home and Everyday Life Settings, and the Role of Laundry. Home Hygiene & Health. International Scientific Forum on Home Hygiene; 2011. p. 47

[39] Bockmühl PD. Hygiene aspects in domestic laundry. Hygiene + Medizin. 2011;**36**:280-286

[40] Stapleton K, Hill K, Day K, Perry DJ, Dean RJ. The potential impact of washing machines on laundry malodour generation. Letters in Applied Microbiology. 2013;**56**:299-306

[41] Nix DI, Frontzek A, Bockmühl PD. Characterization of microbial communities in household washing machines. Tenside, Surfactants, Detergents. 2015;**52**(6):433-440

[42] Butinar L, Strmole T, Gunde-Cimerman N. Relative incidence of ascomycetous yeasts in arctic coastal environments. Microbial Ecology. 2011;**61**(4):832-843. DOI: 10.1007/s00248-010-9794-3

[43] NSF. The Public Health and Safety Organization. International Household Germ Study [Internet]. 2013. Available from: https://www.nsf.org/newsroom_pdf/2013_germ_study_FOR-WEB-ONLY.pdf [Accessed: November 21, 2016]

[44] Catellani P, Miotti Scapin R, Alberghini L, Radu IL, Giaccone V. Levels of microbial contamination of domestic refrigerators in Italy. Food Control. 2014;**42**:257-262

[45] Altunatmaz SS, Issa G, Aydin A. Detection of airborne psychrotrophic bacteria and fungi in food storage refrigerators. Brazilian Journal of Microbiology. 2012;**43**:1436-1443

[46] Enger L, Joly S, Pujol C, Simonson P, Pfaller M, Soll DR. Cloning and characterization of a complex DNA fingerprinting probe for *Candida parapsilosis*. Journal of Clinical Microbiology. 2001;**39**:658-669

[47] Roy B, Meyer SA. Confirmation of the distinct genotype groups within the form species *Candida parapsilosis*. Journal of Clinical Microbiology. 1998;**36**:216-218

[48] Tavanti A, Hensgens LA, Ghelardi E, Campa M, Senesi S. Genotyping of *Candida orthopsilosis* clinical isolates by amplification fragment length polymorphism reveals genetic diversity among independent isolates and strain maintenance within patients. Journal of Clinical Microbiology. 2007;**45**:1455-1462

[49] Tavanti A, Davidson AD, Gow NA, Maiden MC, Odds FC. *Candida orthopsilosis* and *Candida metapsilosis* spp. nov. to replace *Candida parapsilosis* groups II and III. Journal of Clinical Microbiology. 2005;**43**:284-292

[50] Boekhout T, Kurtzman CP. Principles and methods used in yeast classification and an overview of currently accepted yeast genera. In: Wolf K, editor. Non-conventional Yeasts in Biotechnology. Berlin/Heidelberg: Springer; 1996. pp. 1-81

[51] White TJ, Bruns T, Lee S, Taylor WJ. Amplification and direct sequencing of fungal ribosomal RNA genes for phylogenetics. In: Innis MA, Gelfand DH, Ninsky JJ, White TJ, editors. PCR Protocols: A Guide to Methods and Applications. New York: Academic Press, Inc.; 1990. pp. 315-322

[52] Tamura K, Stecher G, Peterson D, Filipski A, Kumar S. MEGA6: Molecular evolutionary genetics analysis version 6.0. Molecular Biology and Evolution. 2013;**30**:2725-2729

Section 3

Antifungal Compounds

Chapter 6

Thiosulfonates: The Prospective Substances against Fungal Infections

Vira Lubenets, Nataliya Stadnytska, Diana Baranovych, Sofiya Vasylyuk, Olena Karpenko, Viktoriya Havryliak and Volodymyr Novikov

Abstract

The synthesis of new analogs of natural biologically active substances is a promising direction for the development of effective antifungal agents. Thiosulfonic acid esters (thiosulfonates) are the structural analogs of biocidal compounds from garlic, onion, cabbage, cauliflower, etc. More than 1000 thiosulfonates of various structures of the general formula RSO_2SR' were synthesized at the Lviv Polytechnic National University, where their physicochemical properties were characterized. A high antifungal activity of the obtained substances was established in relation to the representatives of fungi of different genera. The thiosulfonates are perspective as basis for the development of effective antifungal means for the modern pharmaceutical, food industry, for the protection of various materials and agricultural products. To increase their effectiveness, antimicrobial compositions based on thiosulfonates and surfactants of microbial origin (biosurfactants) in the form of stable suspensions were developed and studied. It has been established that the use of biosurfactants in the compositions allows the enhancement of the antifungal activity of thiosulfonates and reduction of their active concentration. The possible mechanisms of the joint action of thiosulfonates and biosurfactants on fungal pathogens are proposed.

Keywords: fungal infection, thiosulfonates, biosurfactants, biological activity, pathogens

1. Introduction

Thiosulfonic acids and their esters of the general formula RSO_2SR' are close structural analogs of the natural phytoncides of garlic (*Allium sativum*), onion (*Allium cepa*), various types of cabbage, especially cauliflower [1, 2], and also deep-sea urchin *Echinocardium cordatum* [3]. It is well known that synthetic esters of thiosulfonic acids exhibit a wide range of biological activity that often exceeds the efficiency of natural analogs. Some of these esters are proposed as effective antifungal compounds [4, 5], promising substances for other applications [6–12], preservatives of fruits and vegetables, effective plant protection products, growth regulators, biocidal additives [7, 13–15], insecticides, and radioprotectors [16–19].

IntechOpen

Esters of thiosulfonic acids are effective sulfenilating reagents in organic synthesis [19, 20] and also have valuable properties for solving complex problems of molecular biology and biochemistry [16].

Nowadays, synthesis and investigation of thiosulfoesters are carried out by Japanese [21], American [22], Italian [23], Spanish [17, 24], Korean [25], and Chinese [26] scientists from leading research centers. In Ukraine, for many years, the study on the synthesis and physicochemical and biological properties of thiosulfonic acid esters is carried out at the Lviv Polytechnic National University by the staff of the Department of Technology of Biologically Active Compounds, Pharmacy, and Biotechnology [16, 27]. At the present time, a scientific school has been formed that develops a methodology for research on the synthesis of biologically active compounds of the thiosulfonate structure. During this time more than 1000 compounds of the general structure RSO_2SR' were synthesized:

$$Alk - SO_2 - S - Alk \quad Ar - SO_2 - S - Alk \quad Alk - SO_2 - S - Ar \quad Ar - SO_2 - S - Ar$$

$$cykl - C_5H_9 - SO_2 - S - Alk \quad cykl - C_6H_{11} - SO_2 - S - Alk$$

$$Alk - SO_2 - S - C_5H_9 - cykl \quad Alk - SO_2 - S - C_6H_{11} - cykl$$

Among esters of thiosulfoacids, there are compounds with fungicidal activities against fungi of the genera *Candida*, *Fusarium*, *Mucor*, *Phragmidium*, *Ramularia*, *Penicillium*, *Aspergillus*, *Cladosporium*, *Paecilomyces*, *Phoma*, *Rhizopus*, *Saccharomyces*, *Botrytis*, *Stachybotrys*, *Alternaria*, *Aureobasidium*, *Chaetomium*, *Myrothecium*, *Epidermophyton*, *Trichophyton*, *Microsporum*, *Sclerotinia*, *Monilia*, *Trichoderma*, *Verticillium*, *Pullularia*, *Cryptococcus*, *Trichosporon*, and *Geotrichum* [4–16].

Investigation of esters of thiosulfonic acids began after the isolation of natural antibiotic allicin from the garlic juice, which manifests the antimicrobial activities. Allicin is a low stable allyl ester of allylthiosulfine acid [17]. Esters of thiosulfonic acid, in comparison with esters of thiosulfine acid, are stable compounds; the effectiveness of its antimicrobial activity, in particular, antifungal, is equal to or higher than the activity of thiosulfinates [17].

The antimicrobial activity of esters of thiosulfoacids is closely related to their ability to block the normal metabolism of microorganisms through sulfenylation of thiol groups of their enzymes [28]. It is known that these esters are highly reactive compounds that interact with nucleophiles, electrophiles, and radicals. Nucleophilic substitution reactions occur with breaking of -S-S-bond due to the redistribution of electron density in thiosulfogroup that determines the direction of nucleophile attack [9, 16, 29].

The information in the review about the possibility of practical application of thiosulfonates as antifungal substances is based on published data on its use in the modern pharmaceutical, food, other industries, and agriculture.

2. Protection of agricultural products

Plant-fungal infections cause great economic losses due to the reduction in crop yields during its growing and storage. The loss of crops at all stages of production ranges from 15 to 40%. To solve these problems, esters of thiosulfonic acid can be used because they are characterized by low toxicity and are permitted as preservatives for the food industry [30–34]. The products of their decomposition are environmentally safe, so these substances do not harm the environment [29, 35].

S-esters of thiosulfonic acid are proposed for the prevention and control of agricultural products damage, in particular, fruit and vegetable, as these compounds are capable of inhibiting or eliminating rotting processes [36].

2.1 Effect of thiosulfoesters on microorganisms

The minimal inhibitory concentrations (MIC) against such fungi (*Penicillium* sp., *Aspergillus* sp., *Fusarium* sp., *Rhizopus* sp., *Mucor* sp., *Saccharomyces ellipsoideus*, *Candida albicans*) were determined for alkyl, cycloalkyl, trichloromethyl, aryl, and alkyl-functionalized esters of alkane and cycloalkane thiosulfonic acids (**Table 1**).

#	Substances		MIC, µg/ml						
	R	R'	*A*	*B*	*C*	*D*	*E*	*F*	*G*
1	2	3	4	5	6	7	8	9	10
1		CH_3	1.0	4.0	2,0	20.0	1.0	1.0	0.4
2		C_2H_5	40.0	20.0	20.0	20.0	20.0	20.0	-[a]
3		C_4H_9	10.0	4.0	4/0	20.0	20.0	20.0	-[a]
4		i-C_4H_9	4.0	4.0	4.0	10.0	0	4.0	-[a]
5		CCl_3	2.0	20.0	2.0	20.0	20.0	2.0	2.0
6	CH_3	C_2H_5Cl	20.0	100.0	2.0	100.0	100.0	2.0	-[a]
7		C_2H_4OH	4.0	100.0	4.0	100.0	100.0	4.0	20.0
8		CH_2COOH	20.0	20.0	2.0	100.0	100.0	2.0	-[a]
9		*cycl*- C_5H_9	-[a]	-[a]	2.0	-[a]	10.0	-[a]	0.5
10		*cycl*- C_6H_{11}	-[a]	-[a]	2.0	-[a]	5.0	-[a]	1.0
11		CH_3	20.0	100.0	4.0	100.0	20.0	4.0	4.0
12		C_2H_5	10.0	10.0	10.0	10.0	20.0	-[a]	-[a]
13		C_4H_9	10.0	10.0	10.0	100.0	100.0	-[a]	-[a]
14		C_4H_9-*i3o*	10.0	10.0	10.0	100.0	0	-[a]	-[a]
15		CCl_3	4.0	2.0	2.0	4.0	2.0	2.0	-[a]
16	C_2H_5	C_2H_5Cl	4.0	20.0	2.0	100.0	100.0	2.0	-[a]
17		C_2H_5OH	1.0	20.0	1.0	100.0	20.0	2.0	-[a]
18		CH_2NH_2*HBr	0	0	0	0	0	0	-[a]
19		CH_2COOH	0	0	0	0	0	-[a]	-[a]
20		*cycl*- C_5H_9	-[a]	-[a]	2.0	-[a]	100.0	-[a]	50.0
21		*cycl*- C_6H_{11}	-[a]	-[a]	0.4	-[a]	20.0	-[a]	0.2
22	C_3H_7	*cycl*- C_5H_9	-[a]	-[a]	5.0	-[a]	10.0	-[a]	1.0
23		*cycl*- C_6H_{11}	-[a]	-[a]	0.4	-[a]	100.0	-[a]	0.2
24	C_4H_9	*cycl*- C_5H_9	-[a]	-[a]	5.0	-[a]	50.0	-[a]	1.0
25		*cycl*- C_6H_{11}	-[a]	-[a]	1.0	-[a]	-[a]	-[a]	0.2
26		C_2H_5	4.0	10.0	4,0	40.0	-[a]	10.0	-[a]
27		$CH_2CH(CH_3)_2$	4.0	4.0	4.0	40.0	-[a]	4.0	-[a]
28	$C_6H_5CH_2$	$CH(CH_3)C_2H_5$	4.0	100.0	2.0	100.0	100.0	4.0	-[a]
29		C_2H_5Cl	20.0	20.0	20.0	0	0	-[a]	4.0
30		C_2H_5OH	0	0	100.0	0	0	-[a]	0
31		CH_2COOH	0	0	0	0	0	-[a]	0

Note. # — number of compounds
A: *Penicillium* sp.;B: *Aspergillus* sp.; C: *Fusarium* sp.; D: *Rhizopus* sp.; E: *Mucor* sp.; F: *Saccharomyces ellipsoideus*; G:*Candida albicans*
0 Not activity -[a] Not tested

Table 1.
Minimal inhibitory concentrations of AlkSO$_2$SR' [37].

It has been shown that the fungicidal activity of cyclopentyl (## 9, 20, 22, 24, **Table 1**) and cyclohexyl S-esters of alkanthiosulfonic acids (## 10, 21, 23, 25, **Table 1**) is similar or higher than the activity of alkyl S-esters of alkanthiosulfonic acid (## 1–4, 11–14, **Table 1**), especially for *Fusarium* sp., *Mucor* sp., and *Candida albicans.*

The minimal inhibitory concentration for cyclopentyl S-esters (## 9, 20, 22, 24, **Table 1**) varied from 0.5 to 50.0 μg/ml, and for cyclohexyl S-esters, it was in the range of 0.2–5.0 μg/ml. For cyclohexyl S-esters of alkanthiosulfonic acid (## 10, 21, 23, 25, **Table 1**), the inhibitory concentration is from 0.2 to 2.0 μg/ml relative to *Fusarium* sp., and *Candida albicans* [28, 29]. For cyclohexyl S-esters of alkanthiosulfonic acid (## 10, 21, 23, 25, **Table 1**), the minimal inhibitory concentration ranged from 0.2 to 2.0 μg/ml against *Fusarium* sp. and *Candida albicans* [37, 38].

Among the S-esters of cyclopentane-hexanethiosulfonic acid (## 1–19, **Table 2**) and cyclohexanethiosulfonic acid (## 10–19, **Table 2**), trichloromethyl S-esters (## 4, 13, **Table 2**) are most effective against *Fusarium* sp. and *Candida albicans* but less active against *Mucor* sp. [38].

It has been found that cyclopentyl C_6H_5-SO_2-S-C_6H_{11}-cycl (# 6, **Table 3**) and cyclohexyl C_6H_5-SO_2-S-C_5H_9-cycl (# 3, **Table 3**) S-esters of benzenethiosulfonic acid C_6H_5-SO_2-S-C_6H_{11}-cycl (# 6, **Table 3**) exhibit high activity against *Candida albicans* (MIC 2.0 μg/ml and 1 μg/ml, respectively), *Fusarium avenaceum* (MIC 5.0 μg/ml and 2.0 μg/ml, respectively), and a lower activity against *Mucor* sp. [38].

#	Substances		MIC, μg/ml						
	R	R'	*A*	*B*	C	*D*	*E*	*F*	G
1	2	3	4	5	6	7	8	9	10
1	*cycl*- C_5H_9	CH_3	-[a]	-[a]	1.0	-[a]	4.0	-[a]	4.0
2		C_2H_5	-[a]	-[a]	2.0	-[a]	20.0	-[a]	0.2
3		C_3H_7	-[a]	-[a]	1.0	-[a]	20.0	-[a]	0.4
4		CCl_3	-[a]	-[a]	0.05	-[a]	5,0	-[a]	0.02
5		CH_2CH_2Cl	-[a]	-[a]	5.0	-[a]	50.0	-[a]	1.0
6		CH_2CH_2OH	-[a]	-[a]	20.0	-[a]	200.0	-[a]	20.0
7		CH_2COOH	-[a]	-[a]	50.0	-[a]	50.0	-[a]	5.0
8		C_6H_5	-[a]	-[a]	10.0	-[a]	100.0	-[a]	10.0
9		4-$NO_2C_6H_4$	-[a]	-[a]	50.0	-[a]	200.0	-[a]	20.0
10	*cycl*-C_6H_{11}	CH_3	-[a]	-[a]	2,0	-[a]	5.0	-[a]	2.0
11		C_2H_5	-[a]	-[a]	5.0	-[a]	10.0	-[a]	2.0
12		C_3H_7	-[a]	-[a]	0.4	-[a]	100.0	-[a]	2.0
13		CCl_3	-[a]	-[a]	0.1	-[a]	100.0	-[a]	0.05
14		CH_2CH_2Cl	-[a]	-[a]	1.0	-[a]	20.0	-[a]	0.2
15		CH_2CH_2OH	-[a]	-[a]	20.0	-[a]	100.0	-[a]	20.0
16		CH_2COOH	-[a]	-[a]	4.0	-[a]	100.0	-[a]	50.0
17		C_6H_5	-[a]	-[a]	20.0	-[a]	100.0	-[a]	10.0
18	*cycl*-C_6H_{11}	4-$NO_2C_6H_4$	-[a]	-[a]	100.0	-[a]	200.0	-[a]	20.0
19		4-$CH_3OC_6H_4$	-[a]	-[a]	50.0	-[a]	100.0	-[a]	50.0
Note. # – number of compounds									
A: *Penicillium* sp.; *B:Aspergillus* sp.; *C:Fusarium* sp.; *D:Rhizopus* sp.; *E:Mucor* sp., *F: Saccharomyces ellipsoideus, G:.Candida albicans*									
0 – Not activity; -[a] Not tested									

Table 2.
Minimal inhibitory concentrations of ***cycl****-AlkSO$_2$SR' [38].*

#	Substances		MIC, μg/ml		
	R-	Alk-*cycl*	*Fusarium avenaceum*	*Mucor sp.*	*Candida albicans*
1	2	3	4	5	6
1	4-CH_3O	*cycl*-C_5H_9	20.0	100.0	10.0
2	4-CH_3CONH	*cycl*-C_5H_9	5.0	50.0	2.0
3	H	*cycl*-C_5H_9	5.0	100.0	2.0
4	4-CH_3O	*cycl*-C_6H_{11}	5.0	200.0	5.0
5	4-CH_3CONH	*cycl*-C_6H_{11}	20.0	-[a]	4.0
6	H	*cycl*-C_6H_{11}	2.0	50.0	1.0

Note. # - number of compounds
-[a]. Not tested

Table 3.
Minimal inhibitory concentrations of 4-R-C_6H_4-SO_2-S-Alk-cycl [38].

2.2 Anti-phytopathogenic activities of esters of thiosulfoacids

The prospects for the use of esters of thiosulfonic acid for the control of clamp rot of beet have revealed. The causative agents of clamp rot of beet are phytopathogens *Botrytis cinerea*, *Fusarium betae*, and *Phoma betae*, which cause the loss of root resource during its storage.

These pathogens damage the roots of beet seedlings, cause spotty leaves, and dry rot of root crops, which lead to a decrease in the taste and commodity performance of products. In laboratory conditions, 18 esters of thiosulfoacid were investigated against these phytopathogens (**Table 4**) [39].

#	Substances		MFC, μg/ml		
	R	R'	*Botrytis cinerea*	*Fusarium betae*	*Phoma betae*
1	2	3	4	5	6
1	CH_3	CH_3	200.0	40.0	40.0
2		C_2H_4OH	400.0 mycelium growth	-	-
3		C_2H_4Cl	100.0	200.0	100.0
4	C_2H_5	CH_3	40.0	100.0	400.0
5		C_2H_5	200.0	100.0	40.0
6		C_4H_9	100.0	200.0	40.0
7		CCl_3	4.0	4.0	200.0
8		C_2H_4OH	400.0 mycelium growth		
9	C_3H_7	CH_3	100.0	40.0	200.0
10		C_3H_7	100.0	100.0	40.0
11		CCl_3	4.0	10.0	400.0
12		CH_2CH_2Cl	400.0	—	—
13	C_4H_9	CH_3	200.0	—	—
14	C_6H_5	CH_3	100.0	40.0	200.0
15	C_6H_5	i-C_3H_7	400.0	—	—
16	4-$CH_3CONHC_6H_4$	C_2H_5	400.0 mycelium growth	—	—
17	$NH_2C_6H_4$	C_2H_5	400.0 mycelium growth	—	—
18	*β*-$C_{10}H_7$	CCl_3	40.0	—	—

Note. # –number of compounds

Table 4.
Minimal fungicidal concentrations of RSO_2SR' against pathogens of clamp rot [39].

The highest efficacy against *Botrytis cinerea* and *Fusarium betae* was observed for trichloromethyl S-esters of ethane and propanethiosulfonic acid (# 7, 11, **Table 4**). Trichloromethyl S-ester β-naphthalene thiosulfonic acid is less active among the synthesized trichloromethyl esters. The most effective against *Phoma betae* are methyl S-ester of methanethiosulfonic acid (# 1, **Table 4**), ethyl and butyl S-esters of ethanethiosulfonic acid (# 5, 6, **Table 4**), and propyl ester of propanethio-sulfonic acid [10]. It has been shown that thiosulfoesters (# 1, 7, 11, **Table 4**) at a concentration of 200 μg/ml are toxic to sugar beet (*Beta vulgaris var. saccharifera*) but have fungicidal activity against these phytopathogens.

It is interesting that trichloromethyl S-esters of methane- and propanethiosulfonic acids, as well as methyl S-esters of methanesulfonic acid at a concentration of 200.0 μg/ml, are nontoxic to sugar beet but exhibit a fungicidal effect on the abovementioned phytopathogenic fungi.

Approval in the farm conditions of the trichloromethyl S-ester of propanethiosulfonic acid (# 11 **Table 4**), as well as its mixtures with methyl-S-ester of methanesulfonic acid, revealed its effectiveness for the treatment of sugar beet root crops for prolonged storage. Improvement of the quality parameters of sugar beet after treatment with the synthesized preparations was established.

Thus, the objects of study were the roots of beet of different qualities. Wilted roots on 15%, damaged ones near the head and tail, roots with 3–4% of green mass and 10% of the earth, and healthy clean roots were used in experiments. After 104 days of storage, all samples of beet treated with solutions of these substances had rotten roots in 2.5–4.0 times less than in untreated control.

The effectiveness of the preparations based on the esters of thiosulfonic acid against the causative agents of clamp rot is confirmed by comparative studies of healthy sugar beet with control, where the amount of rotten mass is greater by 9.3 times [39].

The high antifungal activity of alkyl and trichloromethyl esters of methane-, ethane-, and propanethiosulfonic acids in experiments in vitro was discovered. These data indicate that these compounds can be used for the prevention of fruits and vegetables against fungal damage during prolonged storage. Effective fungicidal concentrations of synthesized nine esters of alkanthiosulfonic acid were found for 13 genera of fungi (**Table 5**):

$$\mathbf{C_2H_5SO_2SR''}\ (\#2c, 2e),\quad \mathbf{RSO_2SCH_3}\ (\#1a, 2a, 3a),\quad \mathbf{RSO_2SCl_3}\ (\#1b, 2\,b, 2d, 3b)$$

The highest fungicidal activity of trichloromethyl esters was found at concentrations of 40–1.25 μg/ml, while alkyl esters of alkanthiosulfonic acids exhibit fungicidal activity at concentrations of 5–100 μg/ml against fungi of the genera *Fusarium*, *Rhizopus*, and *Mucor*, which in some cases is higher than for trichloromethyl esters [40].

The antifungal activity of some alkyl and trichloromethyl esters of aromatic thiosulfonic acids as preservatives for protecting fruits and vegetables during storage against fungal damage was also studied (**Table 6**) [40].

The positive effect was observed after the use of 4-aminophenyl ester of 4-aminobenzenesulfonic acid (# 2a, **Table 6**) to prevent potato rot during storage. It is significant that this ester is less toxic than alkyl esters of alkanthiosulfonic acid. The potato was treated with a solution of this substance at concentrations of 40 and 20 μg/ml (at a rate of 100 ml or 4–8 mg of dry substance per 1 ton of potatoes). After 1.5 months storage, the amount of potato waste decreased by 2.5 times. The ability of some esters of thiosulfonic acids to protect tomatoes from fungal damage during storage was also studied. The most active and low toxic were the ethyl

#	Fungi	MFC of substances, μg/ml								
		1a	1b	2a	2b	2c	2d	2e	3a	3b
1	2	3	4	5	6	7	8	9	10	11
1	*Penicillium glaucum*	40.0	10.0	40.0	10.0	10.0	10.0	20.0	10.0	1.67
2	*Penicillium expansum*	40.0	1.25	40.0	5.0	5.0	1.25	—	10.0	1.67
3	*Penicillium digitatum*	20.0	5.0	20.0	10.0	5.0	5.0	10.0	20.0	2.5
4	*Penicillium italicum*	20.0	10.0	40.0	10.0	10.0	40,0	10.0	20.0	1.67
5	*Aspergillus niger*	20.0	2.5	40.0	10.0	10.0	20.0	—	40.0	2.5
6	*Fusarium solani*	20.0	80.0	20.0	10.0	10.0	40.0	20.0	40.0	20.0
7	*Fusarium moniliforme*	20.0	40.0	20.0	10.0	10.0	40.0	10.0	20.0	40.0
8	*Rhizopus nigricans*	80.0	100.0	80.0	5.0	100.0	180.0	10.0	80.0	20.0
9	*Mucor racemosus*	20.0	40.0	20.0	10.0	10.0	20.0	20.0	40.0	20.0
10	*Botrytis cinerea*	40.0	1.67	20.0	20.0	20.0	5.0	40.0	40.0	1.67
11	*Botrytis allii*	20.0	20.0	50.0	10.0	20.0	20.0	40.0	20.0	2.5
12	*Sclerotinia* sp.	40.0	10.0	10.0	40.0	20.0	10.0	20.0	20.0	20.0
13	*Monilia fructigena*	40.0	20.0	80.0	20.0	50.0	20.0	40.0	40.0	10.0

Note. # – number of compounds
1a: R=CH_3, R'=CH_3; 1b: R=CH_3, R'=CCl_3;
2a: R=C_2H_5, R'= CH_3; 2b: R=C_2H_5, R'= CCl_3; 2c: R=C_2H_5, R'= C_4H_9; 2d: R=C_2H_5, R'= CCl_3;
2e: R=C_2H_5, R'=C_6H_5
3a: R= C_3H_7, R'=CH_3; 3b: R= C_3H_7, R'=CCl_3

Table 5.
Minimal fungicidal concentrations of RSO_2SR' for the prevention of fruits and vegetables [40].

#	Funges	MFC of substances, μg/ml		
		1a	1b	2a
1	2	3	4	5
1	*Penicillium glaucum*	10.0	2.5	10.0
2	*Penicillium expansum*	5.0	1.25	-
3	*Penicillium digitatum*	5.0	5.0	10.0
4	*Penicillium italicum*	20.0	10.0	5.0
5	*Aspergillus niger*	40.0	2.5	-
6	*Fusarium solani*	20.0	2.5	10.0
7	*Fusarium moniliforme*	20.0	20.0	10.0
8	*Rhizopus nigricans*	180.0	80.0	2.5
9	*Mucor racemosus*	20.0	10.0	5.0
10	*Botrytis cinerea*	40.0	1.67	5.0
11	*Botrytis allii*	20.0	20.0	20.0
12	*Sclerotinia* sp.	40.0	10.0	5.0
13	*Monilia fructigena*	40.0	20.0	20.0

Note. # — number of compounds
1a: R=HR'=CH_3; 1b: R=H, R'=$CCl_3$2a: R=NH_2, R'=4-$NH_2C_6H_4$

Table 6.
Minimal fungicidal concentrations of 4-$RC_6H_4SO_2SR'$ for the prevention of fruits and vegetables [40].

esters of 4-acetylamino- and 4-aminobenzenethiosulfonic acids. It was established that the treatment of tomatoes by these preparations in laboratory conditions was accompanied by a significant decrease in the amount of waste after 10–12 days of storage.

The effectiveness of alkyl esters of 4-aminobenzenethiosulfonic acids against phytopathogens—the causative agents of citrus fruits' damage—was studied. Citrus fruits were purchased in the Ukrainian trade networks (Lviv). Mycelial fungi *Ramularia chelidonii* and *Phragmidium fragariae* were isolated and identified as pathogens, which cause the damage of lemons and mandarins. It has been shown that isolated cultures exhibit middle and high sensitivity to all studied esters (**Table 7**). Growth inhibition zones of isolated microorganisms at concentrations of active substances of 0.5% and 1% were on average 25–30 mm [41].

In experiments, the ability of S-ethyl ester of 4-aminobenzenethiosulfoacid (ETS) to elicit an antifungal effect against pathogens of fruit and vegetable damage was tested. Minimal inhibitory and minimal fungicidal concentrations against four genera of fungi *Aspergillus*, *Penicillium*, *Paecilomyces*, and *Cladosporium* by methods of diffusion and serial dilutions at a microbial load of 5×10^5 CFU/ml were determined (**Table 8**) [41].

2.3 Effect of Propyl propanethiosulfinate and Propyl propanethiosulfonate on phytopathogens

Propyl propanethiosulfinate (PTS), $C_3H_7SOSC_3H_7$, and propylpropylthiosulfonate (PTSO), $C_3H_7SO_2SC_3H_7$, isolated from garlic (*Allium sativum L.*) and onion (*Allium cepa L.*) were proposed by the Spanish researches for the prevention and control of fungal diseases of plants, for crop storage and as disinfectants for food industry, and for the sanitary treatment of cold rooms, equipment, fruit packaging, and vegetables. PTS and PTSO can be used both in pure form and in the form of aqueous mixtures or suspensions with other synthetic or natural antifungal agents, fertilizers, antioxidants, and plant growth regulators. These compounds can be used in different ways such as immersion, wetting, spraying, applying to soil, etc. [17].

The results, presented in **Table 9**, indicate that PTSO is more active compound against *Penicillium solitum* (wild-type strain) than less stable PTS.

These substances are effective protection agents of tomatoes, peppers, cucumbers, melons, lettuce, stone fruits, citrus fruits, strawberries, tropical fruits like avocado, and mango against *Pseudoperonospora cubensis*, *Phytophthora infestans*, *Erysiphe* sp., *Sphaerotheca* sp., *Leveillula taurica*, *Botrytis cinerea Pers.*, *Alternaria dauci*, *Alternaria citri*, *Venturia inaequalis*, *Monilia fructicola*, *Monilia laxa*,

#	Compound	Concentration, %	Zones of growth inhibition, mm	
			Phragmidium fragariae	*Ramularia chelidonii*
1	2	3	4	5
1	$NH_2C_6H_4SO_2SC_3H_5$	0.1	21	10
		0.5	27	20
		1.0	30	23
2	$NH_2C_6H_4SO_2SCH_3$	0.1	21	0
		0.5	25	17
		1.0	28	24
3	$NH_2C_6H_4SO_2SC_2H_5$	0.1	19	11
		0.5	24	23
		1.0	26	30

Table 7.
Antifungal activity of $NH_2C_6H_4SO_2SAlk$ [41].

#	Fungi	Method of diffusion, mm		Method of serial dilution	
		Concentration, 0.1 %	Concentration, 0.3 %	MIC, μg/ml	MFC, μg/ml
1	2	3	4	5	6
1	*Aspergillus niger*	0	25.0	125.0	250.0
2	*Aspergillus terreus*	15.0	20.0	62.5	125.0
3	*Aspergillus fungus*	0	22.0	-[a]	-[a]
4	*Penicillium chrysogenum*	20.0	25.0	62.5	62.5
5	*Penicillum* sp.	18.0	20.0	-[a]	-[a]
6	*Paecilomyces variotti*	20.0	20.0	31.2	62.5
7	*Cladosporium resinae*	-[a]	-[a]	15.6	31.2

-[a] Not tested

Table 8.
Antifungal activity of $NH_2C_6H_4SO_2SC_2H_5$ [41].

Microorganisms	PTS, μg/ml					PTSO, μg/ml				
	1000	500	250	125	60	1000	500	250	125	60
1	2	3	4	5	6	7	8	9	10	11
Penicillium solitum wild strain	35	28	16	11	0	40	30	20	12	0
Enterococcus faecalis ATCC 29212	30	30	26	22	15	45	45	45	33	26
Listeria innocua CECT 4030	40	37	32	23	13	52	43	35	20	13

Table 9.
Comparative activities of PTS and PTSO against test-microorganisms [17].

Taphrina deformans, *Phytophthora* spp., *Phytophthora infestans*, *Oidium fragariae*, and *Colletotrichum gloeosporioides* [17], which cause downy mildew, *Botrytis* (gray mold), alternariosis, spotted, powdery mildew, Monilia, bruised, *Alternaria* of citrus fruits, and gummosis.

Pathogens *Penicillium expansum*, *Botrytis cinerea*, *Physalospora obtusa*, *Glomerella cingulata*, and *Botryosphaeria ribis* can cause blue mold, gray mold, black rot, sour rot, and white rot in postharvested apples, pears, and quince [17].

3. Protection of materials against biodamage

A serious problem is the biodamage to various materials and products, which is accompanied by annual economic losses. Therefore, there is a need to find ways to solve problems related to the protection of raw materials and products from the action of causative agents during its prolonged storage, transportation, and operation.

In view of this, S-esters of thiosulfonic acid RSO_2SR can be promising biocides to protect materials and products since they have a wide range of antifungal and antibacterial effects. The sulfonyl and thiol component of S-esters determines their biocidal action spectrum; therefore, it is important to expand the information on the correlation of the dependence of the structure of S-esters of thiosulfonic acids with its useful characteristics [14, 42].

Ninety-three esters of thiosulfonic acids of various structures in relation to the protection of industrial materials (adhesives, wood, paper, textiles, leather, lubricating liquids, paints, and polymer products) against the fungi, yeasts, bacteria, algae, and mucilages were studied by researchers of the concern "Bayer." These compounds are also proposed as biocidal additives in circulating water circuits at industrial plants, in particular, oil refineries [43].

The effectiveness of the synthesized compounds was studied on the following species of fungi: *Alternaria tenuis*, *Aspergillus niger*, *Chaetomium globosum*, *Coniophora puteana*, *Lentinus tigrinus*, *Penicillium glaucum*, *Polyporus versicolor*, *Aureobasidium pullulans*, *Sclerophoma pithyophila*, and *Trichoderma viride.* These thiosulfoesters can be used in various forms: powders, wet powders, suspensions, pastes, soluble powders, dust, and granules [43].

The optimal active concentrations of esters of thiosulfoacids were investigated in the range of 0.001–5.0% by weight. Effective fungicidal concentrations to protection of the materials are ranged within 0.05–1.0% by weight [43].

The minimal inhibitory concentration of some esters against *Penicillium brevicaule* (200 μg/ml), *Chaetomium globosum* (300 μg/ml), and *Aspergillus niger* (400 μg/ml) were determined.

The antifungal effect of S-esters of thiosulfonic acids for the protection of various materials (lubricating liquids, products of the oil refining industry and equipment at profile enterprises) is determined [44, 45].

These substances can be used for biocidal protection and conservation of works of art, library, and archive funds for long-term storage [46].

3.1 Effect of esters of thiosulfonic acids on paper protection from biodamage.

The effectiveness of the paper protection with S-esters of thiosulfonic acids against test-cultures—*Aspergillus niger*, *Penicillium chrysogenum*, and *Candida tenuis*—compared with reference nipagin (methyl ester of 4-hydroxybenzoic acid) was established [47].

Ethyl S-ester 4′-nitrobenzylidene-4-aminobenzenesulfonic acid in a concentration of 0.01% inhibits the growth of test-cultures of mold fungi by 20%, more than nipagin at a concentration of 0.1% [47].

A comparative study of the resistance of the paper treated with solutions of synthesized compounds (S-ethyl-4'-nitrobenzylidene-4-aminobenzenethiosulfonate, a mixture of ethylthiosulfanilate and polyvinylpyrrolidone in a ratio of 1:2, nipagin) was performed at 100% humidity and 28°C for 36 days against test-cultures (*Penicillium chrysogenum* BKMF-245, *Aspergillus niger* BKMF-1119, *Mucor plumbeus* BKPMF-520) and evaluated by conditional score (**Table 10**) [48].

It is interesting that the reference preparation nipagin was less effective against fungal action than thiosulfonates (**Table 10**) [48]. Acetone solutions based on thiosulfonates and their formulations with polyvinylpyrrolidone were developed. Adding polyvinylpyrrolidone improves the physico-mechanical and fungal resistant indices of paper [46, 49].

3.2 Influence of esters of thiosulfonic acids on the protection of the oil and oil refining industry equipment and lubricants from biodegradation

Oil, refined products, and equipment for the oil, oil refining, and petrochemical industries can also be subjected to biological damage. Therefore, the main way to fight the harmful microflora is to use environmentally friendly biocides that violate the enzymatic systems of microorganisms and inhibit its activity [50, 51]. To solve this problem, a nontoxic (LD_{50} = 2000 mg/kg) ethyl S-ester 4-aminobenzenethiosulfonic acid (ETC) biocide was proposed [44]. Comparing the antifungal activity of the ETS with the reference industrial biocide on the basis of water-soluble 1,3,5-tris-(2-hydroxyethyl)-perhydro-1,3,5-triazine, it was found that the reference biocide

Compound	Concentration, %	*Aspergillus niger* BKMF – 1119			*Penicillium chrysogenum* BKMF – 245			*Mucor plumbeus* BKIIMF – 520		
		Duration of experiment, day								
		7	12	36	7	12	36	7	12	36
		Degree of lesion, conditional score								
1	2	3								
n-nitrophenyl-ethylsulfanilate	0.1	0.5	1	1	0	0	0	0	0	0
	0.05	1	2	2	0	0.5	1	0	0.5	0
	0.01	2	3	3	1	1	1	0	1	1
Ethylsulfanilate: polyvinylpyrolidone 1:2	0.1	1	1	1	0	0.5	1	0	0.5	0
	0.05	1.5	2	2.5	0.5	1	1.5	0	1	0.5
	0.01	2	3	3	1	2	2	0.5	2	1
Nipagin	0.1	1	2	3	1	1	2	0.5	1	0.5
	0.05	1.5	3	4	2	2	3	1	2	1
	0.01	2	3	4	3	4	4	1	4	2
control	—	4	5	5	4	5	5	1	5	2
0 – no growth; 0.5 – 5 colonies; 1 – 10 colonies; 2 – 20 colonies; 3 – 40 colonies; 4 – 80 colonies; 5 – more than 100 colonies.										

Table 10.
Fungal resistance of paper, treated by biocides $RC_6H_4SO_2SC_2H_5$ [48].

even at a concentration of 0.15% by weight is noneffective, whereas the effective fungicidal concentration of the ETS is 0.01% by weight (**Table 11**). The MIC and MFC of the ethyl S-ester of 4-aminobenzenethiosulfonic acid are, respectively, 40–160 and 2–160 times lower than those of the reference preparation. The advantage of the ETC is its solubility in organic hydrocarbon compounds, which provides its effect in the total volume of the organic phase of petroleum products.

In addition, the introduction of the ETC into the emulsion reduces the damage to the equipment of the oil and oil refining industry as a result of increasing the corrosion resistance of materials [44].

Experimental and industrial studies have shown the stabilization of the lubricating liquids by the addition of ETC, which increases the usage period of ones. In the control cycle during cold rolling of the metal, the number of microorganisms in lubricating liquids after 6 days was 60 million/ml, that is, 30 times more than in the experimental cycle after using the ETS (2 million/ml).

The ETC improves the physicochemical parameters of lubricating liquids and reduces emulsion consumption and the time to replace the spent emulsion. As a

Fungi	Zones of growth inhibition, mm			MIC, μg/ml	MFC, μg/ml	MIC, μg/ml	MFC, μg/ml
	A		B	A		B	
	0.01%	0.1%	0.15%				
1	2	3	4	5		6	
Aspergillus niger	14	20	0	31.2	62.5	1250	1250
Cladosporium resinae	18	30	0	15.6	31.0	2500	5000
Paecilomyces variotii	17	23	0	62.5	125	5000	5000
Trichoderma viride	15	25	0	62.5	125	2500	5000
A — S- ethyl of 4-amino-benzenethiosulfonic acid; B — 1,3,5-tris- (2-hydroxyethyl) -perhydro-1,3,5-triazine							

Table 11.
Antifungal activity of ethyl ester of 4-amino-benzenethiosulfonic acid and 1,3,5-tris- (2-hydroxyethyl)–perhydro-1,3,5-triazine [44].

whole, productive time of the equipment of enterprises significantly increases. The use of ETC as an antifungal agent for lubricating liquids and emulsion in technological processes creates favorable sanitary and hygienic conditions of work and solves a number of environmental issues [44].

4. The effect of ethylthiosulfanilate on the fungal infections

According to the WHO, more than 20% of the world's population of different age groups is affected by mycoses, especially mycoses of the feet and hands with the damage to the nail plate. The resistance of fungal pathogens to known drugs causes increased mycosis diseases and their complications (secondary infections, allergic reactions, eczema, etc.).

It is well known that ETS exhibits a broad spectrum of antifungal activity against pathogenic fungi [4, 5, 14]. The antifungal effects of ETS against 17 strains of various fungi were studied. It has been found that the MIC of the ETC varies from 3.6 to 500 μg/ml (**Table 12**) and depends on the genus and strain [5, 52].

The causative agents that cause skin and systemic diseases are yeast of the genus *Candida*. The antifungal activity of ETS was determined for the most virulent representatives of *Candida albicans, Candida tropicalis*, and *Candida stellatoidea*. The MIC of ETS for *C. albicans* is 30 μg/ml, *C. tropicalis* 250 μg/ml, and for *C. stellatoidea* 500 μg/ml. ETS is highly effective against *Aspergillus foetidus* and *Acremonium chrysogenum*, MIC of which is 3.6 μg/ml and 62.5 μg/ml, respectively (**Table 12**) [5, 52, 53].

ETC was proposed as an active substance of the antifungal 1% Esulanum ointment after a detailed study of the antimicrobial effects of a number of esters of thiosulfonic acids in S. Ordzhonikidze All-Union Scientific-Research Institute

Fungi	MIC, μg/ml	Citation
1	2	3
Aspergillus terreus	250	*53*
Aspergillus foetidus	3.6	53
Aspergillus niger	500	53
Aspergillus awamory	250	*53*
Aspergillus niger mold	60.0	*5*
Penicillium canescens	250	*53*
Acremonium chrysogenum	62.5	*53*
Trichoderma viride	250	*53*
Trichoderma terricola	500	*53*
Candida albicans	30.0	*5*
Candida tropicalis	250	*53*
Candida stellatoides	500	*53*
Trichophyton gypseum	60.0	*5*
Microsporum lanosum	15.0	*5*
Achorion schoenleinii	30.0	*5*
Actinomycetes sp.	15.0	*5*
Rhizopus nigricans	50.0	*54*

Table 12.
Antifungal activity of $NH_2C_6H_4SO_2SC_2H_5$ [5, 52, 53].

of Pharmaceutical Chemistry (Moscow). This ointment was developed based on doegling oil and intended for the treatment of tinea pedis and other fungal skin diseases [4, 5, 54].

The advantage of the Esulanum ointment is its keratolytic properties, which promotes rapid penetration of the drug in the deep tissue and provides an effective long-term therapeutic effect [5, 54]. The study of antimicrobial activity of 1% Esulanum emulsion ointment in vitro against a number of microorganisms (*Staphylococcus aureus*, *Streptococcus haemolyticus*, *Escherichia coli*, *Salmonella typhosa*, *Flexner's Bacillus dysenteriae*, *Diphtheria bacillus* (strain PW3), *Bacillus pyocyaneus*, *Proteus vulgaris*, *Anthrax spores*, *Human tubercle bacillus* (H37), *Avian tubercle bacillus*, *Mycobacterium B5*, *Microsporum lanosum*, *Trichophyton gypseum*, *Achorion schoenleinii*, *Actinomycete*s, and fungi *Candida albicans*, *Aspergillus niger*) showed fungicidal properties of the active substance of the ETS. In this case, the MIC and MFC of ETS are practically similar [5].

Clinical studies of the therapeutic effect of 1% ETS ointment in patients with various forms of fungal skin diseases (epidermophytosis, rubrophytosis, microsporia, and trichophytosis) and different clinical manifestations have proven their effectiveness. Based on these results, an instruction for the application of 1% ETC ointment (Esulanum) was developed by the Pharmacological Committee of the Ministry of Health of the former USSR [5].

Experimental part production of 1% Esulanum was introduced into medical practice, but taking into account that the basis of the dosage form was doegling oil, which resources were limited, industrial production was not realized.

The study of the qualitative and quantitative composition of the dosage form based on the ETS and its therapeutic effects is ongoing. The dynamics of the death of *C. tropicalis* cells affected by fungicidal concentrations of the ETS on the model system, similar to human organism processes (37°C), using a microorganism suspension with a cell load of 4×10^5 cells/ml, were detected. It has been found that the minimum fungicidal concentration for cells is 250 μg/ml [52]. Thus, the fungicidal effect of the ETS on *C. tropicalis* is founded after 30 min of exposure (9.09%) and after an hour by 98.48%, and the full therapeutic effect is achieved after 6 h of exposure.

Adding ETS in fungicidal concentrations to the growth medium changes the morphogenesis of *C. tropicalis.* Bumps and fractures appear on the surface of yeast cells, and their manifestation depends on the time of exposure [52]. ETC affects the metabolism of *C. tropicalis*, suppressing endogenous respiration by 87% and the decrease in nucleic acid pool in pathogen cells to 27.52% for DNA and up to 39.13% for RNA. Significant differences were observed in *C. tropicalis* lipogenesis under the influence of this biocide. Thus, subfungicidal concentration of ETS reduces the concentration of almost all classes of phospholipids in cells but increases in the content of lysophosphatidylcholine by 16.25% and phosphatidylcholine by 11.11% [52].

The ETC at fungistatic and subfungicidal concentrations exhibits a membranotropic effect and provides a high degree of co-operability of the membrane structural transitions of cells [55, 56]. The functional state of cell membranes of *C. tropicalis* was assessed by the release of low molecular nucleotide component from cells (pyrimidine and purine bases) under the action of various concentrations of the ETS. Detection of substances at $\lambda = 260$ nm is a sensitive test that characterizes the state of the barrier permeability of the membrane and can be used to study the kinetics of this process.

The obtained results showed that the release of low molecular nucleotide components from *C. tropicalis* begins immediately after the adding of ETS into the medium (*C. tropicalis* cells concentration, 10^6 cells/ ml). The increase of output of purine and pyrimidine-containing compounds from the cell in 4.8 times compared to reference cells was observed, changing the concentration of ETS from 0 to 62.5 μg/ml. The concentration of ETS in the range of 62.5–125 μg/ml causes almost complete loss of these compounds' pool.

The increase in the permeability of *C. tropicalis* membranes under the influence of different concentrations of the ETS or different time of its exposure can be related to high saturation of cell membranes by lipids. The change in permeability of membranes under the action of ETC is probably due to their dynamic structure.

Interaction of ETS and the surface structures of the cell initiate deep structural rearrangements of membranes, which results in increased permeability and, possibly, inhibition of one's physiological functions.

The obtained data suggest that the mechanism of action of the ETS may be related to the disruption of the cytoplasmic membrane, which will lead to significant defects in the delivery of nutrient components to cells and the removal of vital metabolites from them.

So, summing up our results, it can be considered that the mechanism of ETS effects can be related to the disruption of the cytoplasmic membrane that leads to significant defects in the flow of nutrients into the cells and the removal of metabolites from ones [55].

5. Compositions of esters of thiosulfoacids and biosurfactants and their effects on microorganisms

Alkyl esters of alkane- and arene-thiosulfonic acids are hydrophobic compounds, since they are poorly soluble in water, which limits their use as antimicrobial agents. In addition, the surfaces of microbial cells provide the protective barrier to antimicrobials. To increase the solubility and bioavailability of the thiosulfonates, substances that are capable of their solubilization are used, in particular, surface-active substances (surfactants), which can be used as components of ointments, gels, and creams. The most promising ones are biogenic surfactants—products of microbial synthesis (biosurfactants) [57, 58]. Vasileva-Tonkova et al. [59] and Sotirova (2012) described the permeabilizing effect of biosurfactants. They can interact with membrane phospholipids, influence cell hydrophobicity, and have emulsifying ability [53, 59].

The formation of the supramolecular complexes of rhamnolipids with model membrane phospholipids is considered as a possible molecular mechanism of membranothropic action of the biosurfactant, which was shown by electrospray ionization mass spectrometry [60]. These complexes can affect the liquid-crystalline state of the lipid matrix of microbial membranes and change some membrane processes such as cells transport [61].

The permeabilization of cell membranes with surfactants can overcome the barriers and increase the efficacy of various antimicrobial agents. In this regard, biosurfactants can play a significant role as additives in the development of pharmaceuticals due to their ability to enhance solubility or bioavailability of poorly soluble substances [58].

A new promising approach to the creation of effective antimicrobials is proposed, which consists in a synergistic combination of thiosulfonic esters, ethylthiosulfanilate (ETS) or methylthiosulfanilate (MTS), with the biosurfactants of *Pseudomonas* sp. PS-17 strain—rhamnolipid biocomplex (RBC) and rhamnolipids (RL). The introduction of biosurfactants into the compositions allowed the reduction of the active concentrations of thiosulfonates in the resulting products. The antimicrobial potential of compositions based on ETS and MTS with RL was investigated against model strains of various genera and taxonomic groups,

Microorganisms	Zones of growth inhibition, mm					
	0,1 %		0,5 %		1,0 %	
	ETS	ETS + RBC	ETS	ETS + RBC	ETS	ETS + RBC
1	2	3	4	5	6	7
Aspergillus niger	40	50	40	55	48	65
Candida lipolytica	18	30	23	35	33	38
Bacillus mesentericus	17	20	20	23	22	24
Escherichia coli	20	24	25	28	28	31

Note: ETS — ethylthiosulfanilate, RBC — rhamnolipid biocomplex.
RBC was used in concentration 0,01 %; the mixture of polyethylene glycols (PEG 400 and PEG 500) was used as a base for the ointment compositions

Table 13.
Influence of the contents of ointment compositions on the growth of microorganisms [54].

capable of causing damages to human health, agriculture, industrial products, as well as phytopathogens. So, for culture *Rhizopus nigricans*, MFCs for MTS, 30 μg/ml, and for ETS, 50 μg/ml, and for their compositions RL were, respectively, 10 and 20 μg/ml [53, 60].

The explanation of these results could be related to permeabilization of the microbial cell membranes by rhamnolipids (increase in levels of extracellular proteins). Biosurfactants provoke changes in cell surface and affect different components of the membranes [62]. Biosurfactant also can damage the surface structure of the spores [53, 63].

The developed ointment composition exhibits high antifungal and antibacterial activity in comparison with known biocidal agents. The addition of rhamnolipid biosurfactants into thiosulfonate compositions contributed to the decrease of minimal fungicidal and bactericidal concentrations [53, 64]. The criteria for selecting the ratios of ETS and RBC in the compositions were the formation of stable emulsions and the antifungal and antibacterial activity of the compositions. Comparative studies of the effectiveness of ointment preparations based on ETC and the composition of ETS + RBC with respect to microorganisms of various taxonomic groups were carried out (**Table 13**).

Thus, the presence of the biosurfactant enhanced the biocidal effect of MTS and ETS. A possible explanation could be related to the higher protein leakage as a result of permeabilization with the rhamnolipid biosurfactant. Probably, the decrease in concentrations of the studied substances, which are able to suppress the microbial growth completely, is due to the increased access of inhibitors to the bacterial cell. The use of rhamnolipids or other biosurfactants active against variety of microorganisms, in combination with antibiotic treatment, or antimicrobials, may represent new productive antimicrobial strategy [65].

6. Antifungal activity of various esters of carboxylic and heterocyclic thiosulfonic acids

The series of alkyl-, cycloalkyl- and aryl-esters of arylthiosulfonic acids $RNHC_6H_4SO_2SR'$ was synthesized, and the spectrum of their antifungal action was studied (**Table 14**) [27].

For $RNHC_6H_4SO_2SR'$ (**Table 14**), MIC was determined for *Candida albicans* ATCC 90028, *Candida glabrata* ATCC 90030, *Aspergillus fumigatus* IHEM 13934, and MFC for *Candida albicans*, *Verticillium dahliae*, *Trichophyton gypseum*. All synthesized esters are characterized by rather high fungicidal activity. The compounds

#	Compound		MIC, μg/ml			MFC, μg/ml		
	R	R'	A.	B	C	D	*E*	*F*
1	2	3	4	5	6	7	8	9
1	CH_3CO	CH_3	50.0	-[a]	25.0	100.0	40.0	20.0
2		C_2H_5	25.0	-[a]	12.5	40.0	40.0	10.0
3		C_3H_5	100.0	-[a]	12.5	-[a]	-[a]	-[a]
1		3	4	5	6	7	8	9
4	CH_3CO	C_4H_9	-[a]	-[a]	-[a]	20.0	10.0	10.0
5		cycl-C_5H_9	-[a]	-[a]	-[a]	2.0	-[a]	-[a]
6		cycl-C_6H_{11}	-[a]	-[a]	-[a]	4.0	-[a]	-[a]
7		C_6H_5	-[a]	-[a]	-[a]	10.0	2.0	4.0
8		C_6H_4Cl-p	-[a]	-[a]	-[a]	10.0	4.0	20.0
9		$C_6H_4NO_2$-o	-[a]	-[a]	-[a]	-[a]	400.0	40.0
10	F_3CCO	CH_3	50.0	100.0	25.0	-[a]	-[a]	-[a]
11		C_2H_5	50.0	50.0	25.0	-[a]	-[a]	-[a]
12	ClC_2H_4CO	CH_3	-[a]	-[a]	-[a]	40.0	40.0	-[a]
13		C_3H_7	-[a]	-[a]	-[a]	400.0	200.0	200.0
14		i-C_3H_7	-[a]	-[a]	-[a]	200.0	-[a]	-[a]
15		C_4H_9	-[a]	-[a]	-[a]	400.0	-[a]	-[a]
16		C_6H_5	-[a]	-[a]	-[a]	40.0	10.0	10.0
17		C_6H_4Cl-p	-[a]	-[a]	-[a]	200.0	200.0	100.0
18		$C_6H_4NO_2$-p	-[a]	-[a]	-[a]	200.0	100.0	200.0

Note. # - number of compounds
[a] Not tested

A: Candida albicans ATCC 90028; B: Candida glabrata ATCC90030; C: Aspergillus fumigatus IHEM 13934; D: Candida albicans; E: Verticillium dahliae; F: Trichophyton gypseum

Table 14.
Minimal inhibitory and fungicidal concentrations of substances of structure $RNHC_6H_4SO_2SR'$ [27].

with an acetyl fragment exhibit a higher fungicidal activity than compounds with a 3-chloropropionyl or trifluoroacetyl fragments. The MIC of ethyl ester of 4-acetylaminobenzenethiosulfonic acid relative to *C. albicans* is 25 μg/ml and for fungi *A. fumigatus*, 12.5 μg/ml, while the MIC of the ethyl ester of 4-trifluoroacetyl aminobenzenethiosulfonic acid was, respectively, 50 and 25 μg/ml. Regarding the influence of substituents (R') from the side of sulfide sulfur, cycloalkyl- and aryl thiosulfone esters were more active than alkylic. The MFC values of phenyl esters of 4-acetyl and 3-chloropropionyl aminobenzenethiosulfonic acids were determined between 2–10 and 10–40 μg/ml, respectively.

The evaluation of the fungistatic effect of methyl, ethyl, and allyl esters of 3-acetylamino-4-methoxybenzenethiosulfonic on test-cultures of *C. albicans* and *Penicillium* sp. with an exposure time of 24–120 h was conducted [64]. At a concentration of 200 μg/ml methyl and allyl esters partially delay growth at exposure for 24 h. With an exposure of 48 h at a concentration of 100 μg/ml, allyl ester completely inhibits the growth of *C. albicans*, which is associated with a change in the antifungal mechanism [66].

People with reduced immunity are often exposed to disease, provoked by fungal infections. It was established that alkyl esters of alkane and arylthiosulfonic acids, alkyl esters of heterocyclic thiosulfonic acids have high antifungal activity. MIC of alkyl esters of 2,3-dioxo-1,2,3,4-tetrahydroquinoxaline-6-thiosulfonic acid was established for various fungal strains of *Candida*, *Cryptococcus*, *Trichosporon*, and *Geotrichum* [67–71]. For fungi of the genus *Candida*, the most effective is the allyl ester (C_3H_5) (**Table 15**).

Fungi	MIC [μg/ml]					
	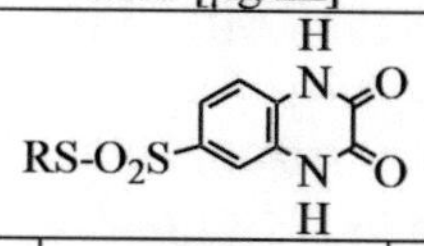					
	CH_3		C_2H_5		C_3H_5	
	24h	48h	24h	48h	24h	48h
1	2	3	4	5	6	7
C. albicans ATCC 90028	25.0	25.0	50.0	50.0	10.0	10.0
C. tropicalis ATCC 750	25.0	50.0	12.5	50.0	25.0	50.0
C. parapsilosis ATCC 90018	100.0	100.0	<6.25	25.0	6.25	25.0
C. krusei ATCC 6258	25.0	50.0	25.0	50.0	10.0	10.0
C. inconspicua IHEM 15763	25.0	25.0	12.5	12.5	25.0	25.0
C. norvegensis IHEM 19639	25.0	50.0	25.0	50.0	12.5	25.0
C. kefyr IHEM 15765	25.0	50.0	50.0	100.0	50.0	100.0
C. lusitaniae IHEM 3979	-	12.5	-	100.0	-	25.0
C. glabrata ATCC 90030	100.0	>100.0	25.0	100.0	25.0	100.0

Table 15.
Fungicidal action of alkyl esters of 2,3-dioxo-1,2,3,4-tetrahydroquinoxaline-6-thiosulfonic acid against Candida sp. [67].

Strain	MIC [μg/ml]								
	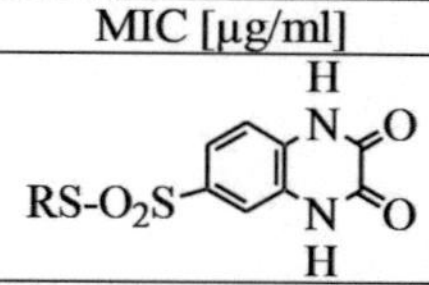								
	CH_3			C_2H_5			C_3H_5		
	48 h	72 h	96 h	48 h	72 h	96 h	48 h	72 h	96 h
1	2	3	4	5	6	7	8	9	10
Cryptococcus neoformans IHEM 14227	<6.25	12.5	-[a]	25.0	50.0	-[a]	6.25	12.5	-[a]
Cryptococcus neoformans IHEM 3969	-[a]	<6.25	6.25	-[a]	25.0	50.0	-[a]	<6.25	12.5
Trichosporon asahii IHEM 17912	<6.25	<6.25	-[a]	25.0	25.0	-[a]	<6.25	12.5	-[a]
Geotrichum capitatum Lab1969	12.5	25.0	-[a]	12.5	25.0	-[a]	<6.25	6.25	-[a]
Geotrichum capitatum Lab1967	-[a]	-[a]	<6.25	-[a]	-[a]	12.5	-[a]	-[a]	<6.25
[a]Not tested									

Table 16.
Fungicidal action of alkyl esters of 2,3-dioxo-1,2,3,4-tetrahydroquinoxaline-6-thiosulfonic acid against Cryptococcus, Trichosporon, and Geotrichum [67].

This regularity is characteristic to fungi of genera *Cryptococcus*, *Trichosporon*, and *Geotrichum* (**Table 16**).

The fungistatic effect of methyl, ethyl, and allyl esters of 8-quinolinethiosulfonic acid on the test-culture of *C. albicans* exposed during 24–120 h was evaluated. For all investigated esters, the inhibitory concentration is 200 μg/ml. Ethyl and allyl esters are more active and their MIC is 100 μg/ml. At a concentration of 1.0 μg/ml, the ethyl ester partially delay the growth of the test-culture exposed for 24–48 h [70, 71].

Summing up our results of the antimicrobial activity of esters of thiosulfonic acids, various ways of their practical application can be proposed. It has been shown that there is a correlation between the structure of thiosulfonate esters, their reactivity in chemical and biochemical reactions, and biological activity. This is confirmed by the specificity of the effects of thiosulfonates against various pathogenic fungi, depending on the structure of their sulfenyl and thiol components.

Our finding showed the advantages of synthetic esters of thiosulfonic acids in comparison with their natural analogs by the biological activity, as well as their competitiveness compared with commercial antifungal substances. The competitiveness of thiosulfonates is determined by their low fungicidal and bactericidal concentrations and low resistance of microorganisms to their action.

Thus, new thiosulfoacid esters as biologically active compounds are suitable for the development of more efficient and safe medicines, biocides, remedies, and growth stimulators.

Author details

Vira Lubenets[1]*, Nataliya Stadnytska[1], Diana Baranovych[1], Sofiya Vasylyuk[1], Olena Karpenko[2], Viktoriya Havryliak[1] and Volodymyr Novikov[1]

1 Lviv Polytechnic National University, Lviv, Ukraine

2 Department of Physical Chemistry of Fossil Fuels InPOCC, L. M. Lytvynenko InPOCC, NAS of Ukraine, Lviv, Ukraine

*Address all correspondence to: vlubenets@gmail.com

References

[1] Nakamura Y, Matsuo T, Shimoi K, Nakamura Y, Tomita I. S-methyl methanethiosulfonate, a new antimutagenic compound isolated from *Brassica oleracea* L. *var. Botrytis*. Biological & Pharmaceutical Bulletin. 1993;**16**:207-209. DOI: 10.1248/bpb.16.207

[2] Benkeblia N, Lanzott V. Allium thiosulfinates: Chemistry, biological properties and their potential utilization in food preservation. Food - Global Science Book. 2007;**1**(2):193-201

[3] Takada N, Watanabe M, Suenaga K, Yamada K, Kita M, Uemura D. Isolation and structures of hedathiosulfoniscasids A and B, novel thiosulfonic acids from the deep-sea urchin *Echinocardium cordatum*. Tetrahedron Letters. 2001;**42**:6557-6560. DOI: 10.1016/S0040-4039(01)01314-4

[4] Boldyirev BG, Kolmakova LE, Pershin GM, Milovanova SN, Pozharskaya AM. i dr: Esulan – novoe sredstvo dlya lecheniya epidermofitii stop. Khymyko-farmatsevtycheskyi zhurnal. 1968;**2**(4):12-16. (In Russian)

[5] Pershin GN, Kukushkina TS, Guskova TA. Esulan. Khimiko-Farmatsevticheskii Zhurnal. 1976;**10**(11):146-150. (In Russian)

[6] Bernard S, Yves B, Henri D (Frantslya). MKI S 07 D 235/28; A 61K 31/47/Nouveaux derives thiosulfonates, leur procede de preparation ainsi que les compositions pharmaceutiques les contenant; № 8417286; Zayavlen. November 13, 84; Opubl. May 16, 86; RZhH. 9O138P. Patent 2573077 Frantslya

[7] Benkeblia N, Lanzotti V. Allium thiosulfinates: Chemistry, biological properties and their potential utilization in food preservation. Food - Global Science Books. 2007;**1**(2):193-201

[8] Gabriele E, Ricci CM, Eneghetti F, Ferri N, Asai A, Sparatore A. Methanethiosulfonate derivatives as ligands of the STAT3-SH2 domain. Journal of Enzyme Inhibition and Medicinal Chemistry. 2017;**32**(1):337-344. DOI: 10.1080/14756366.2016.1252757

[9] Smith M, Hunter R, Stellenboom N, Kusza DA, Parker MI, Hammouda ANH, et al. The cytotoxicity of garlic-related disulphides and thiosulfonates in WHCO1 oesophageal cancer cells is dependent on S-thiolation and not production of ROS. Biochimica et Biophysica Acta. 2016;**1860**:1439-1449. DOI: 10.1016/j.bbagen.2016.03.032

[10] Foskolos A, Siurana A, Rodriquez-Prado M, Ferret A, Bravo D, Calsamiglia S. The effects of a garlic oil chemical compound, propyl-propane thiosulfonate, on ruminal fermentation and fatty acid outflow in a dual-flow continuous culture system. Journal of Dairy Science. 2015;**98**(8):5482-5549. DOI: 10.3168/jds.2014-8674

[11] Fleischauer AT, Arab L. Garlic and cancer: A critical review of the epidemiologic literature. The Journal of Nutrition. 2001;**3S**:1032S-1040S. DOI: 10.1093/jn/131.3.1032S

[12] Perrino E, Cappelletti G, Tazzari V, Giavini E, Del Soldato P, Sparatore A. New sulfurated derivatives of valproic acid with enhanced histone deacetylase inhibitory activity. Bioorganic & Medicinal Chemistry Letters. 2008;**18**:1893-1897. DOI: 10.1016/j.bmcl.2008.02.007

[13] Shvets V, Karpenko O, Karpenko I, Novikov V, Lubenets V. Antimicrobial action of compositions based on thiosulfonates and biosurfactants on phytopathogens. Innovative Biosystems and Bioengineering. 2017;**1**(1):43-48

[14] Boldarev BG, Bilozor TK, Vlyazlo RI, Kozharskiy AI, Lubenets VI, Luzhetskaya OV, et al. Protivomikrobnaya i fiziologicheskaya aktivnost efirov tiosulfo-kislot i vozmozhnyie puti ih prakticheskogo ispolzovaniya v razlichnyih otraslyah narodnogo hozyaystva. Biopovrezhdeniya v promyishlennosti. Mezhvuzovskiy sbornik. — Gorkiy, izdatelstvo Gorkovskogo gosudarstvennogo universiteta, 1983:44-51. (In Russian)

[15] Peinado MJ, Ruiz R, Echávarri A, Rubio LA. Garlic: Derivative propyl propane thiosulfonate is effective against broiler enteropathogens in vivo. Poultry Science. 2012;**91**(9):2148-2157. DOI: 10.3382/ps.2012-02280

[16] Lubenets VI. Tiosulfonaty: syntez i vlastyvosti. Ukrainskii Khimicheskii Zhurnal. 2003;**69**(3):109-117. (in Ukrainian)

[17] Garcia-Pareja MP, Sanchez-Vaquero E, Ayala EG, Lopez FM, Alhendin (Granada). Use of antimicrobial agents derived from alliaceous plants for the prevention and control of crop diseases, post-harvest rot and as environmental disinfectant products. Appl. No.: 12/219,136; Filed: July 11, 2008; Pub. Date: January 15, 2009. Patent 2009/0018194A1 US

[18] Dos Santos EA, Gonçalves FM, Prado PC, Sasaki DY, de Lima DP, Macedo ML. Synthesis method for thiosulfonate and report of its insecticidal activity in *Anagasta kuehniella* (*Lepidoptera: Pyralidae*). International Journal of Molecular Sciences. 2012;**13**(11):15241-15251. DOI: 10.3390/ijms131115241

[19] Reeves B, Hilmer J, Mellmann L, Hartzheim M, Poffenberger K, Johnson K, et al. Selective trapping of SNO-BSA and GSNO by benzenesulfinic acid sodium salt: Mechanistic study of thiosulfonate formation and feasibility as a protein S-nitrosothiol detection strategy. Tetrahedron Letters. 2013;**54**:5707-5710. DOI: 10.1016/j.tetlet.2013.08.011

[20] Trost BM. Alpha-sulphenylated carbonyl compounds in organic synthesis. Chemical Reviews. 1978;**78**:363-382. DOI: 10.1021/cr60314a002

[21] Taniguchi N. Copper-catalyzed synthesis of thiosulfonates by oxidative coupling of thiols with sodium sulfinates. European Journal of Organic Chemistry. 2014;**26**:5691-5694. DOI: 10.1002/ejoc.201402847

[22] Rathnayaka H, Mozziconacci O, Sreedhara A, Schoneich C. Fragmentation of a monoclonal antibody by peroxotungstate. Pharmaceutical Research. 2018;**35**(11):1-15

[23] Gabriele E, Brambilla D, Ricci C, Regazzoni L, Taguchi K, Ferri N, et al. New sulfurated derivatives of cinnamic acids and rosmaricine as inhibitors of STAT3 and NF-β transcription factors. Journal of Enzyme Inhibition and Medicinal Chemistry. 2017;**32**(1):1012-1028. DOI: 10.1080/14756366.2017.1350658

[24] Abad P, Arroyo-Manzanares N, Garcıa-Campana AM. A rapid and simple UHPLC-ESI-MS/MS method for the screening of propyl propane thiosulfonate, a new additive for animal feed. Analytical Methods. 2016;**8**:3730-3739. DOI: 10.1039/c6ay00219f

[25] Hwang SJ, Shyam PK, Jang H-Y. Synthesis of vinyl sulfones via I2-mediated alkene sulfonylations with thiosulfonates. Bulletin of the Korean Chemical Society. 2018;**39**(4):535-539

[26] Liang C, Luo S-H, Kai J, Wang B-W, Chu-Ming P, Wang Z-Y, et al.

Disproportionate coupling reaction of sodium sulfinates mediated by BF3·OEt2: An approach to symmetrical/unsymmetrical thiosulfonates. Organic Letters. 2018;**20**(16):4754-4758

[27] Lubenets V, Vasylyuk S, Monka N, Bolibrukh K, Komarovska-Porokhnyavets O, Baranovych D, et al. Synthesis and antimicrobial properties of 4-acylaminobenzenethiosulfoacid S-esters. Saudi Pharmaceutical Journal. 2017;**25**:266-274

[28] Pylypets R, Iskra Y, Havryliak VV, Nakonechna AV, Novikov VP, Lubenets VI. Effects of thiosulfonates on the lipid composition of rat tissues. Ukrainian Biochemical Journal. 2017;**89**(6):58-64. http://ukrbiochemjournal.org/2017/12/effects-of-thiosulfonates-on-the-lipid-composition-of-rat-tissues.html

[29] Banya AR, Karpenko OY, Lubenets VI, Baranov VI, Novikov VP, Karpenko OV. Influence of surface-active rhamnolipid biocomplex and ethylthiosulfanilate on growth and biochemical parameters of plants in oil contaminated soil. Biotechnologia Acta. 2015;**8**(5):71-77. DOI: 10.15407/biotech8.05.071

[30] Boldyirev BG, Grim AI, Nikitina KV. Sposob predohraneniya plodov ot porchi pri hranenii B.I. (SSSR) A.s. № 186,274 SSSR; 1966. p. 18. (In Russian)

[31] Allyak IV, Boldyirev BG, Melnichenko EL. Sposob predohraneniya ovoschey ot porchi pri hranenii. (SSSR) A.s. № 186,849 SSSR; 1966. p. 19. (In Russian)

[32] Beltyukova KI, Boldyirev BG. Efiryi tiosulfokislot—Novyie sredstva dlya borbyi s bakterialnyimi boleznyami rasteniy. DAN SSSR. 1957;**117**(3):500-503. (In Russian)

[33] Boldyirev BG, Ayzeman BE, Beltyukova KI, Zelepuha SI. Sposob borbyi s gribkovyimi i bakterialnyimi boleznyami selskohozyaystvennyih kultur i stimulyatsii razvitiya rasteniy. Izobreteniya. Prom. obraztsyi. Tovarnyie znaki. (SSSR) A.s. № 103382 MSH SSSR; 1956. p. 12. (In Russian)

[34] Boldyirev BG, Gar KA, Evteeva NV. Efiry tiosulfokislot novyie fungitsyidnyie sredstva. DAN SSSR 1960;**132**(2):346-348. (In Russian)

[35] Lubenets VI, Vasyliuk SV, Nakonechna AV, Shvets VV, Bania AR, Karpenko OV, et al. Zastosuvannia S-etyl-4-aminobenzentiosul-fonatu yak rehuliatora rostu ta biotsydu dlia borotby z fitopatohennoiu mikrofloroiu pry fitorekultyvatsii naftozabrudnenykh gruntiv. zaiavnyk i vlasnyk NU "Lvivska politekhnika". – № u201707007; zaiavl. 03.07.2017; opubl. 10.04.2018, Biul. №7. Patent UA 124324 S07S381/04 (in Ukrainian)

[36] Lubenets V, Vasylyuk S, Baranovych D, Komarovska O, Rayevska K, Zaichenko O, et al. The plant protection remedies of thiosulfonate type. Chemicals in Agriculture and Environment. 2007;**8**:163-167

[37] Boldarev B, Ayzenman B, Zelepuha S, Shvayger M, Mandrik T. O deystvii efirov tiosulfokislot na bakterii i gribyi. Fiziologicheski aktivnnyie veschestva. Respublikanskiy Mezhvuzovskiy Sbornik. 1973;**5**:24-32. (In Russian)

[38] Ayzenman B, Skorobogatko T, Boldarev B, Aristahova L. O protivomikrobnoy aktivnosti efirov tiosulfokislot - proizvodnyih tsiklopentana i tsiklogeksana. Fiziologicheski aktivnnyie veschestva. Respublikanskiy Mezhvuzovskiy Sbornik. 1975;**7**:113-116. (In Russian)

[39] Helemskiy MZ, Chepegina FD, Boldarev BG. Primenenie efirov tiosulfokislot dlya borbyi s kagatnoy gnilyu. Fiziologicheski aktivnnyie veschestva. Respublikanskiy

Mezhvuzovskiy Sbornik. 1972;**4**:110-113. (In Russian)

[40] Boldarev B, Hrymm A, Nykytyna K. Efiru tyosulfokyslot—Novi konservanty dlia predokhranenyia plodov y ovoshchei ot porchy pry khranenyy Fyzyolohychesky aktyvni veshchestva. Respublykanskyi Mezhvuzovskyi Sbornyk. 1971;**3**:148-154. (In Russian)

[41] Stadnytska N, Shved O, Chervetsova V, Monka N, Lubenets V, Novikov V. Doslidzhennia in vitro tiosulfonativ dlia zakhystu ahroproduktsii vid fitopatoheniv. Zbirka naukovykh prats IX zizdu Ukrainskoho tovarystva henetykiv i selektsioneriv im. M.I. Vavylova "Dosiahnennia i problemy henetyky, selektsii ta biotekhnolohii". Kyiv. Lohos. 2012;**4**:609-612. (in Ukrainian)

[42] Lechado CN, Arjona AB, Ayala EG, Lopez VA, Moll CN, Rus AS. Use of propyl propane thiosulfinate and thiosulfonate for the prevention and reduction of parasites in aquatic animal. Appl. No.: 15/713,840; Filed: August 25, 2017; Date: January 18, 2018. Patent 2018/0014538 A1 US

[43] Kretschik O, Koln DE, Kugler M, Leichlingen DE, Jaetsch T, Koln DE. Thiosulfonic acid S-esters as agents for protecting material. Appl. No.: 10/015,321; Filed: December 12, 2001; Date: October 17, 2002. Patent 2002/0151570 A1 US

[44] Shved OV, Lubenets VI, Baranovych DB, Novikov VP, Yarish MIe. Zastosuvannia S-etyl-4-aminobenzentiosulfonatu yak biotsydu dlia zakhystu naftoproduktiv, metaliv ta obladnannia. № a 2005 04194 zaiav. May 04, 2005; opublik. December 15, 2006. - Biul. № 12. Patent UA 77586. MPK 7 A 01N 29/08, 31/14, 33/06, 33/08, S07S.381/04

[45] Novikov VP, Lubenets VI, Baranovych DB. Biotsyd dlia zakhystu naftoproduktiv ta obladnannia naftopererobnykh pidpryiemstv vid bioposhkodzhen. № 2003042917; Zaiavl. April 03, 2003; Opubl. January 15, 2004.- Biul. № 1. Patent UA 63325 A. UA. MPK 7 A01N29/08. 31/14. 33.00

[46] Kadyliak MS, Komarovska-Porokhniavets OZ, Onyshchenko TI, Shved OV, Novikov VP. Sirkovmisna kompozytsiia dlia zakhystu paperu. MPK (2007) D21H 25/00, A01N 31/00, A01N 25/02, C07C 309/00. U 20031110091 opubl. January 15, 2007, Biul.№2. Patent UA 67615

[47] Komarovska-Porokhniavets O, Hubrii Z, Shved O, Moskalenko N, Iskiv O, Novikov V. Antymikrobni vlastyvosti N-zamishchenykh tiosulfonativ. Visnyk Natsionalnoho Universytetu "Lvivska politekhnika". Khimiia, Tekhnolohiia Rechovyn ta Yikh Zastosuvannia. 2008;**622**:44-46

[48] Kadyliak M, Komarovska-Porokhniavets O, Shved O, Onyshchenko T, Novikov V. Doslidzhennia biotsydiv dlia zakhystu paperu vid bioposhkodzhen. Visnyk Natsionalnoho Universytetu "Lvivska politekhnika". Khimiia, Tekhnolohiia Rechovyn ta Yikh Zastosuvannia. 2004;**497**:71-73

[49] Kadyliak MS, Komarovska-Porokhniavets OZ, Onyshchenko TI, Skorokhoda VI, Suberliak OV, Shved OV, et al. Biotsydna kompozytsiia dlia zakhystu paperu. MPK (2006) D21H 25/00. U 20040503904 opubl. July 17, 2006, Biul.№7. Patent UA 76229

[50] Koval E, Sydorenko L. Mykodestruktory nefteproduktov. Mikodestruktoryi promyishlennyih materialov: nauchnoe izdanie inctituta mikrobiologii i virusologii im. D.K. Zabolotnogo AN USSR. - Kiev: Naukova dumka. 1989:142-171: il. - ISBN 5-12-000779-1. (In Russian)

[51] Lozynskyi M, Kachan V, Hevaza Y, Maskaiev AK. Stan i osnovni

napriamy robit po zakhystu mastylno-okholodzhuiuchykh ridyn vid bioushkodzhen. Visnyk - AN URSR. 1983;**8**:55-58

[52] Starovoitova S, Oriabinska L, Lubenets V. Spectrum antimicrobial action of the original antifungal drug Esulanum. Naukovi visti Natsionalnoho tekhnichnoho universytetu Ukrainy “Kyivskyi politekhnichnyi instytut. 2015;**3**:68-76. (In Ukrainian)

[53] Sotirova A, Avramova T, Stoitsova S, Lazarkevich I, Lubenets V, Karpenko E, et al. The importance of rhamnolipid-biosurfactant-induced changes in bacterial membrane lipids of *Bacillus subtilis* for the antimicrobial activity of thiosulfonates. Current Microbiology. 2012;**65**(19):534-541

[54] Lubenets V, Karpenko O, Ponomarenko M, Zahoriy G, Krychkovska A, Novikov V. Development of new antimicrobial compositions of thiosulfonate structure. Chemistry & Chemical Technology. 2013;**7**:119-124

[55] Oriabinska, Starovoitova S, Vasylyuk S, Novikov V, Lubenets V. Ethylthiosulfanilate effect on *Candida tropicalis*. Ukrainian Biochemical Journal. 2017;**89**(5):70-76

[56] Starovoitova S, Oryabinska L, Lubenets V. Influence of antimycotic esulanum on lipid composition and functions of cytoplasmic membrane of *Candida tropicalis* yeast. Biotechnology and Microbiology. Scientific Works of NUFT. 2015;**21**(3):31-37

[57] Rodrigues L, Teixeira J. Chapter 6: Biomedical and therapeutic applications of biosurfactants. In: Sen R, editor. Biosurfactants. Advances in Experimental Medicine and Biology. Vol. 672. New York, NY: Springer; 2010. pp. 75-78

[58] Bhadoriya S, Madoriya N, Shukla K, Parihar MS. Biosurfactants: A new pharmaceutical additive for solubility enhancement and pharmaceutical development. Biochemical Pharmacology. 2013;**2**:113. DOI: 10.4172/2167-0501.100011

[59] Vasileva-Tonkova E, Galabova D, Karpenko E, Shulga A. Biosurfactant-rhamnolipid effects on yeast cells. Letters in Applied Microbiology. 2001;**33**:280-284

[60] Pashynska V. Mass spectrometric study of rhamnolipid biosurfactants and their interactions with cell membrane phospholipids. Biopolymers and Cell. 2009;**25**(6):504-508

[61] Pashinskaya V, Kosevich M, Gomory A, Lisetski L. Mechanistic investigation of the interaction between bisquaternary antimicrobial agents and phopholipids by liquid secondary ion mass spectrometry and differential scanning calorimetry. Rapid Communications in Mass Spectrometry. 2002;**16**(18):1706-1713

[62] Sotirova A, Spasova D, Vasileva-Tonkova E, Galabova D. Effects of rhamnolipid-biosurfactant on cell surface of *Pseudomonas aeruginosa*. Microbiological Research. 2009;**164**:297-303

[63] Banat I, Franzetti A, Gandolfi I, Bestetti G, Martinotti M, Fracchia L, et al. Microbial biosurfactants production, applications and future potential. Applied Microbiology and Biotechnology. 2010;**87**:427-444. DOI: 10.1007/s00253-010-2589-0

[64] Futami J, Yamada H, Kyuragi G, Yagi K. Thiosulfonate compound, reversible cationization agent for protein and/or peptide, and method for solubilization. Appl. No.: 13/636,789; Filed: March 24, 2011; Date: February 18, 2014. Patent No US 8,653,240 B2

[65] Sotirova A, Avramova T, Lazarkevich I, Lubenets V, Karpenko E, Galabova D. Antimicrobial potential

of selected thiosulfonates-based biocides and biosurfactants against bacteria and fungi. Comptes Rendus de L'Academie Bulgare des Sciences. 2010;**63**(9):1307-1314

[66] Lubenets V, Baranovich D, Lisitsa F, Mel'nik O, Vovk I, Gudz O, et al. Synthesis and antimicrobial activity of 3,4-disubstituted benzenethiosulfonic acid esters. Pharmaceutical Chemistry Journal. 2000;**34**(3):118-121

[67] Nawrot U, Zaczyńska E, Czarny A, Lubenets V, Karpenko E. Aktywność przeciw grzybic zasyntetycznych pochodnych allicyny—Kontynuacja badań. Mikologia Lekarska. 2012;**4**(19):143-146

[68] Lubenets VI, Vasylyuk SV, Novikov VP. Synthesis of S-(3-chloroquinoxalin-2-yl) esters of aliphatic and aromatic thiosulfonic acids. Chemistry of Heterocyclic Compounds. 2005;**41**(12):1547-1548

[69] Lubenets V, Vasyliuk S, Hoi O, But S, Cherneha O, Novikov V. Syntez ta vlastyvosti S-esteriv 2,3-diokso-1,2,3,4-tetrahidrokhinoksalin-6-tiosulfokysloty. Zhurnal Orhanichnoi ta Farmatsevtychnoi Khimii. 2007;**53**(19):56-63

[70] Stadnytska N, Lubenets V, Novikov V, Komarovska O, Vovk N, Kryvoruchko O. Syntez ta biolohichna aktyvnist S-alkil(-8-khinolin)tiosulfonativ. Zhurnal Fiziolohichno Aktyvnykh Rechovyn. 2000;**2**(30):27-30

[71] Baranovych D, Stadnytska N, Komarovska O, Hoi O, Lubenets V, Novikov V. Vyvchennia zalezhnosti biolohichnoi aktyvnosti tiosulfonativ vid kyslotnoi i tiolnoi skladovoi. Visnyk DU "Lvivska politekhnika". Khimiia, Tekhnolohiia Rechovyn ta Yikh Zastosuvannia. 2000;**395**:96-99

Section 4

Biological Control Agents

Chapter 7

Advantageous Fungi against Parasites Transmitted through Soil

José Ángel Hernández Malagón,
Cristiana Filipa Cazapal-Monteiro, Rodrigo Bonilla Quintero,
Antonio Miguel Palomero Salinero, María Isabel Silva Torres,
Mathilde Voinot Messnier, María Vilá Pena,
Ángel Romasanta Blanco, José Pedreira García,
Adolfo Paz Silva, Rita Sánchez-Andrade Fernández
and María Sol Arias Vázquez

Abstract

Although many fungal specimens are responsible for human and/or animal infection, other species are advantageous for preventing the infection by soil-transmitted zoonotic parasites. Infection occurs by the accidental ingestion of parasitic stages (cysts, oocysts, eggs, and larvae), their active penetration through the skin or through direct contact. Numerous species of helminths develop an external phase in the soil where the infective stages are attained, thus mammals become infected when grazing, drinking, or accidentally. Ectoparasites as ticks perform also in the soil the phase from egg to larva. Different soil saprophytic fungi that turn into predatory agents when parasitic stages are near have been isolated and described. These species are capable of destroying the pathogens or irreversibly decreasing their viability, providing thus a very interesting and sustainable tool to reduce environmental contamination by pathogenic agents. In the last year, a profound knowledge on the most appropriate fungal species, together with the proper way to disseminate them, has been acquired.

Keywords: *Mucor circinelloides*, *Duddingtonia flagrans*, parasiticide, soil, STHs, zoonoses

1. Introduction

1.1 Organisms in soil

The definition of soil according to the sciences of the earth and life points to the external part of the earth's crust, which is biologically active and tends to develop on the surface of the rocks emerged by the influence of weather and living beings. It is also frequent that this concept includes a complex set of physical, chemical, and biological elements that make up the natural substrate in which life develops on the surface of the continents. The soil is the habitat of a specific biota of microorganisms (bacteria and fungi), plants, and small animals that constitute the edaphon.

In recent decades, there has been an increasing concern for soil biodiversity, on the basis that the interactions between microorganisms, animals, and plants provide an undoubted benefit to the well-being of mammalian species, including man [1]. This biodiversity conditions both the possibilities of feeding these species, oxygenation, as well as the control of the risk of certain diseases. For these reasons, it is not difficult to understand that soil biodiversity is directly affected by global changes caused by man, especially those related to land use, urbanization, agriculture, deforestation, and desertification, which leads to the logical conclusion that the careful and sustainable use of soils would guarantee their benefits.

Different studies have indicated that exposure to soil microorganisms decreases the prevalence of allergic diseases [2]; taking into account the predictions that around the year 2050 two-thirds of the world population will reside in cities, the stimulation of the immune system by soil organisms will be reduced, and therefore allergy cases will increase.

Other researches highlight the increase in the appearance of bacterial species resistant to most known antibiotics, and the same happens with some parasites, such as helminths. The use of remedies found in the soil, such as certain types of fungi, has not yet come to be considered as a solution to the aforementioned problems. It is interesting to know that some bacteria capable of synthesizing effective antibiotics against *Mycobacterium tuberculosis* have been isolated in the soil [3]. It should also be noted the production of molecules with parasiticide action from fungi [4]. Special mention should be made of the use of some fungal species in the control of certain endoparasites that, once in the soil, complete a series of phases until they reach the infective stage [5]. In recent years, very important achievements have been made in the large-scale production of saprophytic fungal spores that are found in the soil, such as *Mucor circinelloides* or *Duddingtonia flagrans*, filamentous species that are in contact with eggs or larvae of some parasites, respectively. They have the capacity to destroy them or limit their viability [6, 7]. In this way, it is possible to reduce the risk of infection in people, and also in animals that are in pasture.

1.2 Pathogenic organisms transmitted through the soil

Pathogenic organisms belong mainly to five main groups, viruses, bacteria, fungi, and parasites (protozoa, helminths, and ectoparasites) [8]. From an academic and disease control approach, the importance of soil lies in the fact that a significant number of pathogens are found in this habitat, and sometimes they are accidentally ingested by animals and people, causing important disorders. There are some organisms that do not require ingestion, being able to spread their pathogenicity through bites or penetrating the skin.

Table 1 summarizes different examples of pathogens present in the soil. It is important to note that most soil organisms do not constitute a health risk, and pathogenic species represent only a minority. Nor should we forget that some species are opportunistic (*Pseudomonas* and *Enterobacter*) and can cause alterations in mammals, although in the soil they are actually antagonists of root pathogens of some plant species, or can act as growth promoters of some plants and even as decomposers of organic matter [9]. Other pathogens need to develop part of their cycle in the soil, to complete their evolution until the infective phase. These are organisms that can survive in the soil for long periods of time, and include spores, eggs, or even larvae. These are obligate pathogens that temporarily reside in the soil, and that are transmitted to mammals by direct contact, by vectors, or through accidental ingestion [10]. For these reasons, it is necessary to know the ecology of

Bacteria	*Bacillus anthracis*	*Agrobacterium tumefaciens*
	Listeria monocytogenes	*Escherichia coli*
	Salmonella spp.	*Clostridium* spp.
Fungi	*Aspergillus* spp.	*Histoplasma capsulatum*
	Coccidioides immitis	
Protozoa	*Naegleria fowleri*	*Toxoplasma gondii*
Helminths	*Ascaris* spp.	*Taenia* spp.
	Ancylostoma spp.	*Strongylus* spp.
Ectoparasites	*Pulex irritans*	*Ixodes* spp.

Table 1.
Numerous pathogens can be found in the soil.

the interactions between the soil and the various organisms to determine why some are prevalent and persist under certain conditions.

The concept of *Soil Borne Human Diseases* offers a very accurate introduction about the role that soil can play in the transmission of certain diseases [11]. However, it is obvious that this idea is a bit limited, since not only the human species will experience the risk of contracting diseases from this habitat. From an etiological point of view, *pathogenic organisms* are defined as those whose habitat is the soil, and *pathogens transmitted by the soil* as organisms that can survive for long periods of time in the soil, and need to do so to infect the host and continue their biological cycle, but they are not part of the soil [12]. Some of the most frequent endoparasites affecting people and animals, such as roundworms, cestodes, or strongyles, belong to this group, and they are characterized by undergoing a series of changes in the soil to the infecting stage. Part of the biological cycle of some ectoparasites such as fleas or ticks occurs in the soil also. This underlines the importance of soil as an adequate medium to certain parasites can survive and develop to infective stages, pending of proper hosts ingest them (flatworms, roundworms, whipworms), contact with soil (hookworms) or walk near (ectoparasites). Regardless of their origin (animal/human), control of parasites affecting mammals requires some action on the stages in the group, since parasiticide therapy acts on the parasites living and affecting them only; thus, the risk of reinfection is elevated, even though successful treatments are applied.

1.3 Mammal parasites developing in the soil

Soil provides a suitable habitat to different organisms as plants can grow and develop, serving as food for the survival of many living creatures (insects and micromammals). This environment enables mammals as herbivores to graze and carnivores to find their feeding.

Most known parasites associated to soil are defined as *soil-transmitted helminths* (STHs), which involve well-known species belonging to flatworms, tapeworms, or roundworms. Helminths can develop a direct cycle in the soil, but an intermediate host is required for some species, and paratenic hosts participate in the transmission of several infections. On the basis of the zoonotic role of different parasites developing in the soil, it is necessary to know the external phase of their life cycle.

Transmission of STHs involves that eggs are passed in the feces of infected individuals. Once in the soil, flatworms (trematodes and cestodes) need to complete several stages inside an intermediate host, to attain the infective stage. *Fasciola hepatica* and *Schistosoma mansoni* (flatworms) are related to humid environments where a number of aquatic or amphibious snails take part. After some stages are completed and exit-off the snails, the infective stages known as metacercariae mature in herbage or water, and infection occurs by the ingestion of herbage or water contaminated [13].

Roundworms (*Ascarids*) represent the most spread nematodes around the world. Although these are host species-specific pathogens, humans can be involved as paratenic hosts for many of them such as roundworms infecting domestic animals (*Toxocara canis*, *Ascaris suum*) or wild species (*Baylisascaris procyonis* and *Toxascaris leonina*). Infection occurs by the accidental ingestion of larvated eggs (containing a second-stage larva inside) (**Figure 1**).

Whipworms (*Trichuris* spp.) have a similar cycle to roundworms. Transmission occurs by the oral ingestion of eggs holding a first larva.

In the case of *Ancylostoma*, nematodes (hookworms), embryonated eggs are passed in the feces and once in the soil, the first-stage larva (L3) emerges and molts to a second-stage larva and then to a third-stage larva, the infective stage. Infection can occur either by oral ingestion of L3 or through the skin [14].

It is well recognized that ticks need to suck blood from mammals for surviving, but sometimes it is forgotten that these ectoparasites develop part of their life cycle in the soil also. Gravid adult females drop off the final host to the ground to lay eggs. Under appropriate conditions, the egg hatches into a larva, which waits for an appropriate mammal to bite for feeding and then transform into nymph.

Appropriate conditions (moisture and temperature) must concur in the soil to improve the development of parasites to their infective stages. Nevertheless, evolution of parasites can be delayed until unfavorable circumstances appear, especially low temperatures. Some of them such as roundworms and whipworms are able to survive viable for long periods, even under temperatures below zero [15]. This

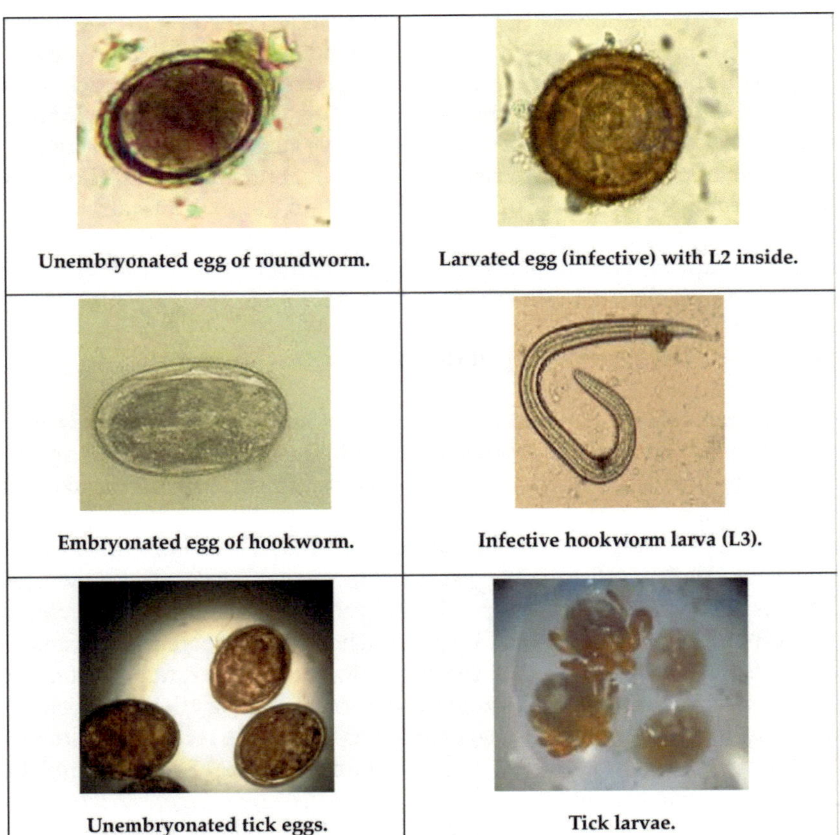

Figure 1.
Numerous parasitic stages can be found in the soil (COPAR archive).

resistance is conferred by their eggshells, composed of at least four layers, uterine (mucopolysaccharides), vitelin, chithinous, and lipidic (inner). Eggs of ticks can also survive in the environment unless the solar light falls directly on them.

Larval stages (first, second, or third) from nematodes exhibit a certain degree of resistance, and it has been reported they can subsist under snowy areas [16]. Dry soils in spite of very humid areas are preferred by immature hookworms [5], like sandy places. This explains the cutaneous infection of people enjoying outdoor activities on beaches, parks, etc. from touristic areas.

1.4 Importance of infection by parasites from the soil

Human STHs are frequent in Asia, Africa, and South America, being absent in Western Europe and developed countries. Nevertheless, these diseases have reemerged due to immigration, travel, and business. Also in recent years, populations of ticks are increasing in urban areas, as well as orchards, parks, and gardens [17].

There are four main STHs affecting humans, *Toxocara canis* (roundworm), *Ancylostoma duodenale* and *Necator americanus* (hookworm), and *Trichuris trichiura* (whipworm). Between 1.5 and 2 billion people, it is believed that they are probably infected worldwide [18]. The presence of these parasites is associated to low standards of hygiene, poverty, and malnutrition because infection takes place by the accidental ingestion of eggs or through cutaneous contact with larvae of hookworms. It is necessary the exposure to feces of pets, mainly dogs. As advised by the WHO (World Health Organization), periodic administration of albendazole and mebendazole is helpful to reduce the incidence of these parasitoses. Deworming is the most applied measure against STHs, and extension of treatment (increment of frequency) looks like a valuable solution, although there is a potential emergence of drug resistance as observed in veterinary medicine [19]. By considering that infections originate from fecal contamination of the environment, mammals can become reinfected frequently after parasiticide treatment is administered. Consequently, actions on the environment are required to reduce the exposure to infective stages, mainly consisting of the use of latrines, together with hygienic behaviors.

Dogs are the definite hosts for *T. canis* and *N. americanus*, thus another question to address concerns the possibility of humans and animals sharing infections by parasites, the so-called parasitic zoonoses. As explained previously, transmission occurs in the same way, but the presence of infected animals becomes essential for human infection. In this case, control appears more difficult, due to the impossibility to ensure that pets receive an appropriate deworming therapy. The problem aggravates when considering that wild/uncontrolled animals can live near persons, because there is no way to perform control of their parasites by the administration of antiparasitic drugs. In some countries, it is not rare to observe feces of stray dogs or cats, foxes or raccoons, in private gardens, public parks, or even beaches. As stated above, humans might become infected by roundworms or hookworms, and despite infection, it is not completed, serious damage could be provoked attributable to the erratic migration of immature stages across the organism [20]. At this point, it seems necessary to remember that second-stage larvae of *Toxocara canis* (dog), *T. cati* (cat), *Ascaris suum* (pig), or *Baylisascaris procyonis* (raccoon) can cause a visceral larva migrans syndrome after these larvae are released at the gut level. Infection by *T. canis* can be responsible for an ocular larva migrans [21], while *B. procyonis* is associated to a devastating neurological syndrome, with children being the riskiest group due to their tendency to play with ground, or take and leave sand in the mouth [22]. The possibility of human infection through the exposure to eggs of roundworms on the coat of dogs has also been considered [23], which remarks the importance of these parasites are easily transmitted to their owners.

2. Beneficial soil fungi

2.1 Antagonists of helminths

By considering that a great number of pathogens develop in the soil, one interesting question refers to why mammals did not infect more frequently, or why low to moderate infections are usually detected. Infection depends on the density of pathogens and risky situations such as accidental ingestion or active passage through the skin (helminths) or walking by places with vegetation (ectoparasites). Then, it could be expected that exposure to natural environments might represent a great hazard, thus enjoying natural habitats should be avoided (or even forbidden).

As mentioned previously, a great number of fungal species can be found in the soil, together with many other organisms such as viruses, bacteria, earthworms, insects, etc. Some of these species are saprophytic and feed on organic matter, but in the presence of parasitic stages such as eggs or larvae, they shift to predatory agents. Hyphae develop and the mycelium grows toward the parasites in an attempt to take certain nutrients, nitrogen and carbon mainly [24]. Other fungal species feed on different species of fungi, as succeeds with some mites.

It has been demonstrated that certain soil saprophytic fungi such as *Duddingtonia flagrans* are able to adapt to the numbers of larvae of nematodes developing from eggs shed in feces of infected grazing horses [25]. In the absence of nutrients, fungi can remain as resting stages (spores). It should be emphasized that different organisms interact simultaneously on the ground, thus soil fungi do not persist for long periods (4 months) and need to be replaced by new structures such as spores, mycelium, etc. [26]. This must be taken into account when soil fungi are going to be used under biological control strategies. Other interesting finding consists of the absence of activity on nonparasitic organisms (**Figure 2**).

Based on experiments with plants, traditionally the fungal antagonists of parasites comprise nematode-trapping species (larvicidal), predacious agents, endoparasitic fungi, and egg parasitic fungi (ovicidal) [27]. In the last decades, this classification applies also for defining the activity of soil fungi against parasites affecting mammals (**Table 2**).

In natural conditions, when the environment does not result altered by humans, soil albeits not only fungi but other microorganisms as viruses, bacteria, earthworms, insects... A number of filamentous fungi feed on organic detritus, certain

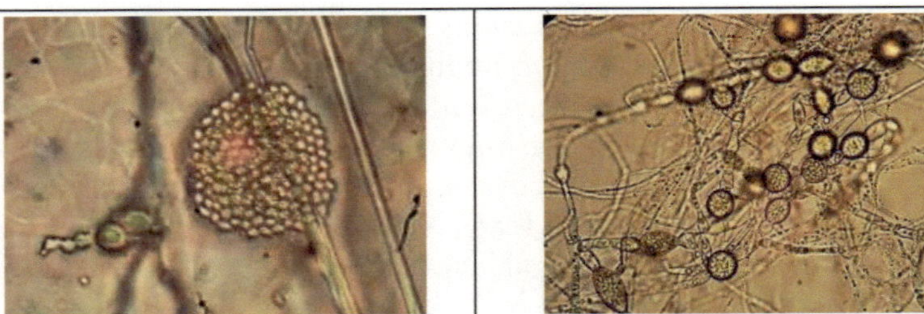

Zygospore of *M. circinelloides*. | Hyphae and chlamydospores of *D. flagrans*.

Figure 2.
Filamentous fungi develop hyphal nets in the soil, and reproduce by spores (COPAR archive).

Effect	Species		Action against
Ovicidal	*Pochonia chlamydosporia*	*Mucor circinelloides*	Flatworms Roundworms (ascarids) Whipworms
	Purpureocillium lilacinus	*Verticillium chlamydosporium*	
	Trichoderma spp.	*Gliocladium* spp.	
Larvicidal	*Duddingtonia flagrans*	*Monacrosporium* spp.	Hookworms Roundworms (strongyles)
	Arthrobotrys spp.		

Table 2.
Filamentous soil fungi antagonists of parasites in the soil.

coprophagous beetles participate in enriching the ground by decomposing organic matter as manure, some mites feed on fungi, and several fungi do it also. This means that an equilibrium situation takes place, where organisms are controlled mutually, and explains also why low risk of infection is usually observed. When agricultural procedures affecting the surface of the ground are performed, this habitat is transformed, and beneficial organisms drop or disappear. As a consequence, the density of pathogens increases, accordingly the risk of exposure among mammals increases and they can become infected.

Several investigations pointed the efficacy provided by some fungi to limit the viability of eggs of roundworms [28]. As drawn in **Figures 3** and **4**, the addition of spores of *M. circinelloides* to the feces of dogs infected by *T. canis* decreased their viability by half after a period of 30 days [29]. When the spores were sprayed onto feces of raccoons parasitized by *B. procyonis*, egg viability reduced by two-thirds also, in agreement with previous experiments [30].

A notable efficacy has been reported against larvae of hookworms by using trapping-nematode fungi such as *D. flagrans*. A 57–73.2% reduction of the numbers of the third-stage larvae of *Ancylostoma* spp. has been obtained, and the counts of larvae decreased by 24.5–63% when exposed to chlamydospores of *D. flagrans* [31, 32].

By taking into account that the aforementioned parasites are STHs, the use of ovicidal and larvicidal fungi could be strongly helpful to limit the development of parasites to infective stages in the soil. One interesting question refers to the proper way to spread the fungi to ensure their contact with the parasites. Because the eggs of parasites are shed by feces, the most useful procedure looks to try that fungi

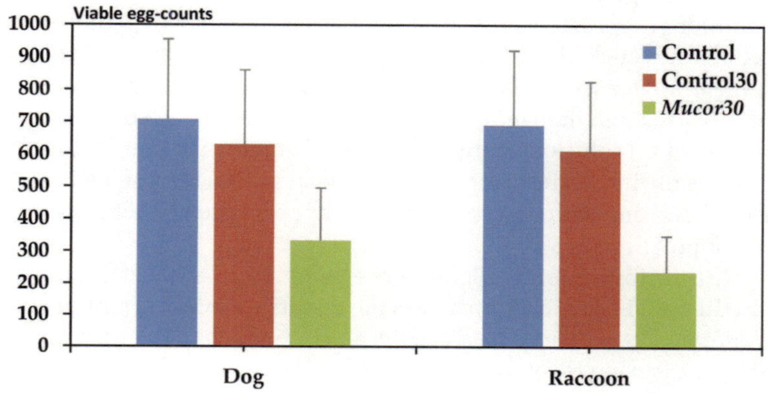

Figure 3.
Viability of eggs of Toxocara canis (left) and Baylisascaris procyonis (right) after 30 days of exposure to spores of Mucor circinelloides (Mucor30) or distilled water (Control 30). Points mean average values and bars the SD [29].

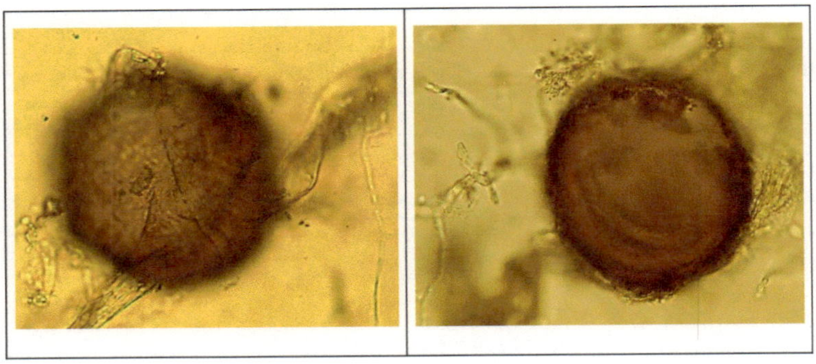

Figure 4.
The soil filamentous fungus M. circinelloides is able to attach to the eggshells of roundworms such as T. canis, colonize, penetrate, and absorb the inner content (COPAR archive).

are in the feces at the same time, and for this purpose, oral administration could be appropriate. Several investigations demonstrated that the spores of *Pochonia chlamydosporia*, *Mucor circinelloides*, and *Duddingtonia flagrans* can survive the passage through the gastrointestinal tract of different animal species, and retained their antagonistic activity [6, 33, 34]. Later, several assays were performed by adding spores or mycelium of *Pochonia chlamydosporia* or *Duddingtonia flagrans* during the handmade elaboration of nutritional pellets [35–37]. More recently, the capability of fungal spores to resist the industrial fabrication of pelleted feed has been demonstrated [38, 39]. The usefulness of pellets containing spores of *M. circinelloides* and *D. flagrans* has been tested on grazing horses, and highly successful results were obtained. Through this strategy, it was possible to reduce the frequency of deworming from 4 years to 1–1.5 years [7, 40]. This approach has also been assayed on wild captive equids maintained in a zoological park, and as a result the administration of anthelmintics was significantly lessened [41], supporting the results previously collected by administering the spores as a premixed feed [6].

2.2 Entomopathological agents

It has been explained that ectoparasites develop part of their cycle in the soil. After mating on the host, gravid female ticks engorge completely and drop to the ground, where thousands of eggs are laid mainly in places protected from sun and desiccation, with vegetation. Later than a variable period, depending on temperature and humidity, eggs hatch and larvae exit off, addressing to plants, pending of a host to attach and suck blood for molting into nymphae. *Beauveria bassiana* and especially *Metarhizium anisopliae* are the most investigated entomopathogenic fungi capable of infecting and damaging ticks [42, 43]. Trials consisted of the topical administration of oil solutions, targeted against immature or adult stages [44]. The aim is to reduce the indiscriminate use of chemical acaricides, for avoiding contamination of food and environment, as well as the appearance of chemical resistance among tick populations [45].

There is little information available concerning the possible effect of fungi on tick eggs in the soil. **Figure 5** summarizes the results collected after the exposure of eggs of *Rhipicephalus boophilus* to spores of *M. circinelloides*. The fungal activity was estimated by measuring the percentage of egg viability, and the hatching percentage, i.e., the percentage of larvae hatched after 15 days. Fungal growth started on the eggshells 4 days after exposure, and by 6 days, hyphae penetrated inside.

Viability of ticks' eggs decreased to 80% in the controls-untreated eggs, and to 38% in those exposed to the filamentous fungus. The hatching percentage was 45% in the controls, by 15% in the *Mucor*-treated eggs.

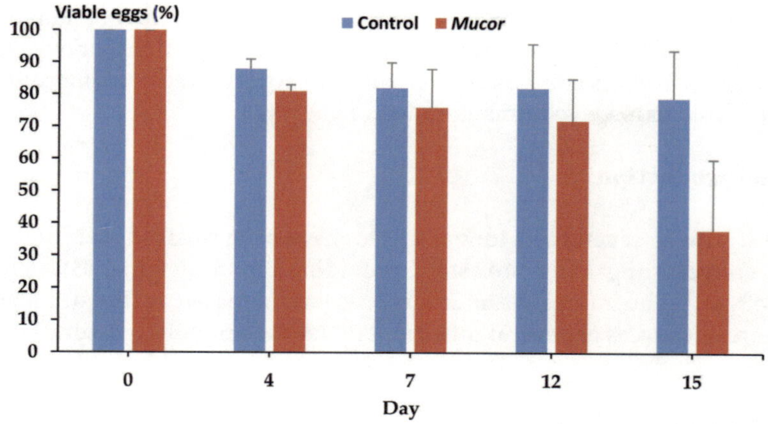

Figure 5.
Viability of eggs of the tick R. boophilus exposed to spores of M. circinelloides (Mucor) or distilled water (Control). Points mean average values and bars the SD (COPAR archive).

Four phases have been described during the activity that the ovicidal fungus *Verticillium chlamydosporium* perform on eggs of helminths, i.e., contact, attachment, penetration, and deliberation [46]. The fungus *M. circinelloides* develops a similar activity on both the eggs of helminths and ticks (**Figure 6**). When the spores contact with the parasites, hyphae grow toward the eggshell and colonize it. Those hyphae facing the eggshell in perpendicular are able to penetrate inside. This is possible due to the involvement of the *appressorium*, a pressing organ consisting of a flattened and thickened hypha, which is provided of a *haustorium*, a specialized branch which penetrates the tissues of the host and absorbs nutrients and water [47]. This mechanism enables the fungus to take all the inner content of the egg, without losing anything. Once completed, hyphae exit off and colonize other egg (deliberation).

In view of the mentioned results, certain soil fungi seem very promising agents for limiting the viability and evolution of tick eggs in the soil, contributing to decrease the risk of infestation. One possible approach could rely on preparing aqueous solutions containing the fungal spores, and spreading by using airless

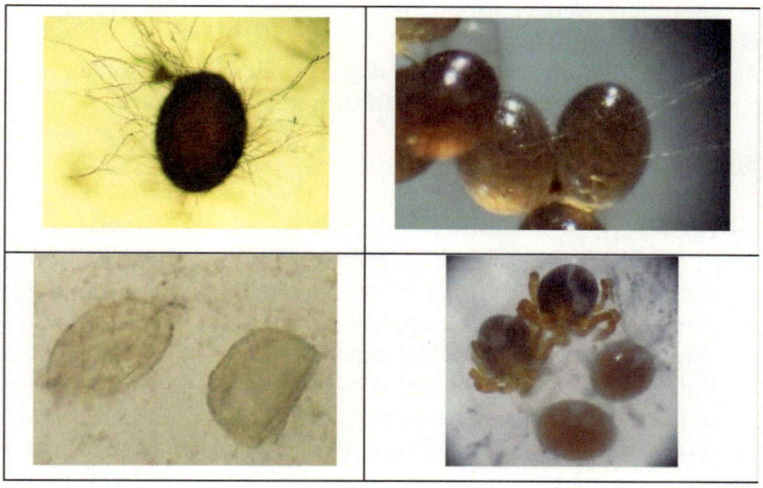

Figure 6.
Hyphae of M. circinelloides grow and attach to the eggshells of ticks, penetrate and destroy them (COPAR archive).

sprayers. This would provide a solution to limit the risk of infestation in outdoor areas as waysides or the edge of grass along the roadsides, gardens, or even farms. Reduction in the presence of ticks in the soil also provides a sustainable and preventive tool to avoid damage to humans and animals.

2.3 Biofuel production

Some strains of several soil fungal species have been isolated according to their ability to convert fungal oils into esters, providing thus a sustainable way to obtain biofuel [48, 49]. The interest of microbial oils has increased as they are now used as commercial sources of several nutritionally important polyunsaturated fatty acids [50].

2.4 Health and soil fungal employment

Despite fungi being mostly considered responsible for fungal diseases that can range from nonsevere to mortal illnesses, fungal infections have become a serious health problem in immunocompromised patients largely.

Opposite to *Duddingtonia flagrans* and *Monacrosporium thaumasium*, the infection by *Mucor circinelloides* has been associated to clinical cases of mucormycosis, a sporadic and life-threatening infection caused by Mucorales. These are fungi distributed far and wide in the environment, in particular on woody surfaces and soils, where it can be easily isolated [27].

Several reports indicated nosocomial infection by *M. circinelloides* among immunocompromised people with skin wounds, or suffering diabetes mellitus [51].

Among animals, infection by *M. circinelloides* has been diagnosed in one Vietnamese potbellied pig presenting clinical signs of pneumonia, but information regarding the habitat or the level of inbreeding has not been provided [52].

Until now, long-term assays comprising the frequent administration (daily or twice a week) of a blend of spores of *M. circinelloides* and *D. flagrans* have been developed in pasturing horses. One group of seven horses received daily pellets containing the fungal spores during 64 weeks, and no adverse effects regarding respiratory, digestive, reproductive, or cutaneous damage were recorded [7]. Other group of eight horses was given pellets twice a week with the spores for a 1-year period, and after testing the activity of the respiratory, digestive, and reproductive systems, no alterations were recorded [41]. No signs of damage on skin integrity were observed.

Until now, there have not been reported any problem with people producing and managing spores/mycelium for longer than 10 years.

2.5 Conclusions

Inasmuch as STHs are transmitted through soil, it seems essential to develop measures on the environment to avoid reinfection, and the abusive administration of parasiticides. Some STHs originate from animals (domestic and wild), and helpful actions to reduce the risk of transmission are also required. Besides public education and hygienic behaviors, other activities should be applied to limit the presence and survival of infective stages of parasites. There have been described several species of soil fungi antagonists of eggs or larvae of helminths and ticks. Although several cases of disease have been linked to soil fungi, the absence of disease among people managing them or among animals receiving fungal structures seems to reinforce their safety, unless the patients are immunocompromised. The use of soil fungi against infections transmitted across ground gives a sustainable measure to prevent damage to persons and animals, and might allow us to limit the administration of antiparasitic drugs to imperative situations only.

Acknowledgements

This work was partly supported by the Research Project CTM2015-65954-R (Ministerio de Economía y Competitividad, Spain; FEDER). Dr. María Sol Arias Vázquez is recipient of a Ramón y Cajal contract (Spanish Ministry of Economy and Competitiveness), and Dr. C.F. Cazapal-Monteiro is beneficiary of a postdoctoral research fellowship (Xunta de Galicia, Spain).

Conflict of interest

All authors declare the absence of any financial or personal interests that could inappropriately influence or bias the current work. The final chapter has been approved by all the authors.

Author details

José Ángel Hernández Malagón, Cristiana Filipa Cazapal-Monteiro, Rodrigo Bonilla Quintero, Antonio Miguel Palomero Salinero, María Isabel Silva Torres, Mathilde Voinot Messnier, María Vilá Pena, Ángel Romasanta Blanco, José Pedreira García, Adolfo Paz Silva*, Rita Sánchez-Andrade Fernández and María Sol Arias Vázquez
COPAR (Control of Parasites) Research Group, Zoonoses and Public Health, Animal Pathology Department, Faculty of Veterinary, University of Santiago de Compostela, Spain

*Address all correspondence to: adolfo.paz@usc.es

References

[1] Bardgett RD, van der Putten WH. Belowground biodiversity and ecosystem functioning. Nature. 2014;**515**:505-511

[2] Hanski I, von Hertzen L, Fyhrquist N, Koskinen K, Torppa K, Laatikainen T, et al. Environmental biodiversity, human microbiota, and allergy are interrelated. Proceedings of the National Academy of Sciences of the United States of America. 2012;**109**:8334-8339

[3] Ling LL, Schneider T, Peoples AJ, Spoering AL, Engels I, Conlon BP, et al. A new antibiotic kills pathogens without detectable resistance. Nature. 2015;**517**:455-459

[4] Hegedüs N, Marx F. Antifungal proteins: More than antimicrobials? Fungal Biology Reviews. 2013;**26**:132-145

[5] Arias MS, Cazapal-Monteiro CF, Suárez J, Miguélez S, Francisco I, Arroyo FL, et al. Mixed production of filamentous fungal spores for preventing soil-transmitted helminth zoonoses: A preliminary analysis. BioMed Research International. 2013;**2013**:567876. DOI: 10.1155/2013/567876

[6] Arias MS, Cazapal-Monteiro C, Valderrábano E, Miguélez S, Rois JL, López-Arellano ME, et al. A preliminary study of the biological control of strongyles affecting equids in a zoological park. Journal of Equine Veterinary Science. 2013;**33**:1115-1120

[7] Hernández JÁ, Arroyo FL, Suárez J, Cazapal-Monteiro CF, Romasanta Á, López-Arellano ME, et al. Feeding horses with industrially manufactured pellets with fungal spores to promote nematode integrated control. Veterinary Parasitology. 2016;**229**:37-44

[8] Janeway CA Jr, Travers P, Walport M, Shlomchik MJ. Immunobiology: The Immune System in Health and Disease. 5th ed. New York: Garland Science; 2001

[9] Berg G, Eberl L, Hartmann A. The rhizosphere as a reservoir for opportunistic human pathogenic bacteria. Environmental Microbiology. 2005;**7**:1673-1685

[10] Brevik EC, Sauer TJ. The past, present, and future of soils and human health studies. The Soil. 2015;**1**:35-46

[11] Jeffery S, van der Putten WH. Soil Borne Human Diseases. JRC Scientific and Technical Reports; 2011. http://publications.jrc.ec.europa.eu/repository/bitstream/111111111/22432/2/lbna24893enn.pdf [Accessed: March 01, 2018]

[12] Wall DH, Nielsen UN, Six J. Soil biodiversity and human health. Nature. 2015;**528**:69-76

[13] Cwiklinski K, O'Neill SM, Donnelly S, Dalton JP. A prospective view of animal and human Fasciolosis. Parasite Immunology. 2016;**38**:558-568

[14] Kwon I, Kim H, Lee J, Choi M, Chai J, Nakamura-Uchiyama F, et al. A serologically diagnosed human case of cutaneous larva migrans caused by *Ancylostoma caninum*. Korean Journal of Parasitology. 2003;**41**:233-237

[15] Jensen PK, Phuc PD, Konradsen F, Klank LT, Dalsgaard A. Survival of *Ascaris* eggs and hygienic quality of human excreta in Vietnamese composting latrines. Environmental Health. 2009;**8**:57

[16] Kuzmina TA. Contamination of the environment by strongylid (Nematoda: Strongylidae) infective

larvae at horse farms of various types in Ukraine. Parasitology Research. 2012;**110**:1665-1674

[17] Michalik J, Hofman T, Buczek A, Skoracki M, Sikora B. *Borrelia burgdorferi s.l.* in *Ixodes ricinus* (Acari: Ixodidae) ticks collected from vegetation and small rodents in recreational areas of the city of Poznań. Journal of Medical Entomology. 2003;**40**:690-697

[18] Dunn JC, Turner HC, Tun A, Anderson RM. Epidemiological surveys of, and research on, soil-transmitted helminths in Southeast Asia: A systematic review. Parasites & Vectors. 2016;**9**:31. DOI: 10.1186/s13071-016-1310-2

[19] Tchuem Tchuenté LA. Control of soil-transmitted helminths in sub-Saharan Africa: Diagnosis, drug efficacy concerns and challenges. Acta Tropica. 2011;**120**(Suppl 1):S4-S11

[20] Chen J, Liu Q, Liu GH, Zheng WB, Hong SJ, Sugiyama H, et al. Toxocariasis: A silent threat with a progressive public health impact. Infectious Diseases of Poverty. 2018;7:59. DOI: 10.1186/s40249-018-0437-0

[21] Liu J, Li S, Deng G, Yang W, Chen W, Lu H. Ultrasound biomicroscopic imaging in paediatric ocular toxocariasis. British Journal of Ophthalmology. 2017;**101**:1514-1517

[22] Błaszkowska J, Góralska K, Wójcik A, Kurnatowski P, Szwabe K. Presence of *Toxocara* spp. eggs in children's recreation areas with varying degrees of access for animals. Annals of Agricultural and Environmental Medicine. 2015;**22**:23-27

[23] Roddie G, Stafford P, Holland C, Wolfe A. Contamination of dog hair with eggs of *Toxocara canis*. Veterinary Parasitology. 2008;**152**:85-93

[24] Casas-Flores S, Herrera-Estrella A. Antagonism of plant parasitic nematodes by fungi. In: Kubicek C, Druzhinina I, editors. Environmental and Microbial Relationships. The Mycota. Vol. 4. Berlin, Heidelberg: Springer; 2007

[25] Paz-Silva A, Francisco I, Valero-Coss RO, Cortiñas FJ, Sánchez JA, Francisco R, et al. Ability of the fungus *Duddingtonia flagrans* to adapt to the cyathostomin egg-output by spreading chlamydospores. Veterinary Parasitology. 2011;**179**:277-282

[26] Saumell CA, Fernández AS, Echevarria F, Gonçalves I, Iglesias L, Sagües MF, et al. Lack of negative effects of the biological control agent *Duddingtonia flagrans* on soil nematodes and other nematophagous fungi. Journal of Helminthology. 2016;**90**:706-711

[27] Hernández JA, Vázquez-Ruiz RA, Cazapal-Monteiro CF, Valderrábano E, Arroyo FL, Francisco I, et al. Isolation of ovicidal fungi from fecal samples of captive animals maintained in a zoological park. Journal of Fungi (Basel). 2017;**3**. DOI: 10.3390/jof3020029

[28] Cortiñas FJ, Cazapal-Monteiro CF, Hernández JA, Arroyo FL, Miguélez S, Suárez J, et al. Potential use of *Mucor circinelloides* for the biological control of certain helminths affecting livestock reared in a care farm. Biocontrol Science and Technology. 2015;**25**:1443-1452

[29] Hernández JÁ. Posibilidades de control de helmintozoonosis por ascáridos mediante el uso de hongos telúricos [thesis]. Spain: University of Santiago de Compostela; 2014. (Spanish)

[30] Cazapal-Monteiro CF, Hernández JA, Arroyo FL, Miguélez S, Romasanta Á, Paz-Silva A, et al. Analysis of the effect of soil saprophytic fungi on the eggs of *Baylisascaris procyonis*. Parasitology Research. 2015;**114**:2443-2450

[31] Maciel AS, Freitas LG, Campos AK, Lopes EA, Araújo JV. The biological control of *Ancylostoma* spp. dog infective larvae by *Duddingtonia flagrans* in a soil microcosm. Veterinary Parasitology. 2010;**173**:262-270

[32] De Mello IN, Braga FR, Monteiro TS, Freitas LG, Araujo JM, Soares FE, et al. Biological control of infective larvae of *Ancylostoma* spp. in beach sand. Revista Iberoamericana de Micología. 2014;**31**:114-118

[33] Casillas Aguilar JA, Mendoza de Gives P, López-Arellano ME, Liébano Hernández E. Evaluation of multinutritional pellets containing *Duddingtonia flagrans* chlamydospore for the control of ovine haemonchosis. Annals of the New York Academy of Sciences. 2008;**1149**:161-163

[34] Braga FR, Araújo JV, Silva AR, Carvalho RO, Araujo JM, Ferreira SR, et al. Viability of the nematophagous fungus *Pochonia chlamydosporia* after passage through the gastrointestinal tract of horses. Veterinary Parasitology. 2010;**168**:264-268

[35] Dias AS, Araújo JV, Braga FR, Araujo JM, Puppin AC, Fernandes FM, et al. Biological control of *Fasciola hepatica* eggs with the *Pochonia chlamydosporia* fungus after passing through the cattle gastrointestinal tract. Parasitology Research. 2012;**110**:663-667

[36] Tavela Ade O, de Araújo JV, Braga FR, da Silveira WF, Dornelas e Silva VH, Carretta Júnior M, et al. Coadministration of sodium alginate pellets containing the fungi *Duddingtonia flagrans* and *Monacrosporium thaumasium* on cyathostomin infective larvae after passing through the gastrointestinal tract of horses. Research in Veterinary Science. 2013;**94**:568-572

[37] Fitz-Aranda JA, Mendoza-de-Gives P, Torres-Acosta JF, Liébano-Hernández E, López-Arellano ME, Sandoval-Castro CA, et al. *Duddingtonia flagrans* chlamydospores in nutritional pellets: Effect of storage time and conditions on the trapping ability against *Haemonchus contortus* larvae. Journal of Helminthology. 2015;**89**:13-18

[38] Arroyo FL, Arias MS, Cazapal-Monteiro CF, Hernández JÁ, Suárez J, Miguélez S, et al. The capability of the fungus *Mucor circinelloides* to maintain parasiticidal activity afer the industrial feed pelleting enhances the possibilities of biological control of livestock parasites. Biological Control. 2016;**92**:38-44

[39] Arias MS, Arroyo FL, Cazapal-Monteiro C, Hernández JÁ, Suárez J, Francisco I, et al. Formulating *Duddingtonia flagrans* in nutritional pellets for the sustainable control of equine strongyles. Journal of Science, Technology and Environment. 2015;**5**(1): Article ID 3000249, 16 pages. ISSN: 2227-9296

[40] Hernández JÁ, Sánchez-Andrade R, Cazapal-Monteiro CF, Arroyo FL, Sanchís JM, Paz-Silva A, et al. A combined effort to avoid strongyle infection in horses in an oceanic climate region: Rotational grazing and parasiticidal fungi. Parasites & Vectors. 2018;**11**:240. DOI: 10.1186/s13071-018-2827-3

[41] Palomero AM, Hernández JA, Cazapal-Monteiro CF, Balán FA, Silva MI, Paz-Silva A, et al. Implementation of biological control to the integrated control of strongyle infection among wild captive equids in a zoological park. BioMed Research International. 2018;**2018**:4267683. DOI: 10.1155/2018/4267683

[42] Camargo MG, Nogueira MR, Marciano AF, Perinotto WM, Coutinho-Rodrigues CJ, Scott FB, et al. *Metarhizium anisopliae* for controlling *Rhipicephalus microplus* ticks under field

conditions. Veterinary Parasitology. 2016;**223**:38-42

[43] Aw KMS, Hue SM. Mode of infection of *Metarhizium* spp. fungus and their potential as biological control agents. Journal of Fungi (Basel). 2017;**3**:E30. DOI: 10.3390/jof3020030

[44] Prado-Rebolledo OF, Molina-Ochoa J, Lezama-Gutiérrez R, García-Márquez LJ, Minchaca-Llerenas YB, Morales-Barrera E, et al. Effect of *Metarhizium anisopliae* (Ascomycete), Cypermethrin, and D-Limonene, alone and combined, on larval mortality of *Rhipicephalus sanguineus* (Acari: Ixodidae). Journal of Medical Entomology. 2017;**54**:1323-1327

[45] Camargo MG, Golo PS, Angelo IC, Perinotto WM, Sá FA, Quinelato S, et al. Effect of oil-based formulations of acaripathogenic fungi to control *Rhipicephalus microplus* ticks under laboratory conditions. Veterinary Parasitology. 2012;**188**:140-147

[46] Lýsek H, Krajci D. Penetration of ovicidal fungus *Verticillium chlamydosporium* through the *Ascaris lumbricoides* egg-shells. Folia Parasitologica. 1987;**34**:57-60

[47] Yoshida S, Cui S, Ichihashi Y, Shirasu K. The haustorium, a specialized invasive organ in parasitic plants. Annual Review of Plant Biology. 2016;**67**:643-667

[48] Carvalho AK, Rivaldi JD, Barbosa JC, de Castro HF. Biosynthesis, characterization and enzymatic transesterification of single cell oil of *Mucor circinelloides*—A sustainable pathway for biofuel production. Bioresource Technology. 2015;**181**:47-53

[49] Szczęsna-Antczak M, Struszczyk-Świta K, Rzyska M, Szeląg J, Stańczyk Ł, Antczak T. Oil accumulation and in situ trans/esterification by lipolytic fungal biomass. Bioresource Technology. 2018;**265**:110-118

[50] Tang X, Zhao L, Chen H, Chen YQ, Chen W, Song Y, et al. Complete genome sequence of a high lipid-producing strain of mucor circinelloides WJ11 and comparative genome analysis with a low lipid-producing strain CBS 277.49. PLoS One. 2015;**10**:e0137543

[51] Garcia-Hermoso D, Criscuolo A, Lee SC, Legrand M, Chaouat M, Denis B, et al. Outbreak of invasive wound mucormycosis in a burn unit due to multiple strains of *Mucor circinelloides f. circinelloides* resolved by whole-genome sequencing. MBio. 2018;**9**:e00573-e00518

[52] Evans DE, Kawabata A, Wilson LD, Kim K, Dehghanpir SD, Gaunt SD, et al. Entomophthoromycosis and mucormycosis as causes of pneumonia in Vietnamese potbellied pigs. Journal of Veterinary Diagnostic Investigation. 2018;**30**:161-164